I AM WITH YOU

I AM WITH YOU

LOVE LETTERS TO CANCER PATIENTS

Blessings. . . .

Nancy Novack

Edited by Nancy Novack, Ph.D.
and Barbara K. Richardson

For information, write to:
Nancy's List Books
www.NancysList.org
Nancy@NancysList.org

Cover design by Jake Messing, *www.jakemessing.com*
Interior design by Corrin Acome, *www.corrinacome.com*
Cover photograph by Linda Schreyer

Library of Congress Cataloging-in-Publication Data

I am with you : love letters to cancer patients / edited by Nancy
Novack and Barbara K. Richardson ; written by and for amazing
cancer patients everywhere.
    pages cm
  ISBN 978-0-692-42200-7
1. Cancer—Patients—Biography. 2. Cancer—Patients—Psychology.
3. Cancer—Patients—Correspondence. I. Novack, Nancy (Clinical
psychologist) II. Richardson, Barbara K., editor,
  RC265.5.I3 2015
  362.19699'400922--dc23
                        2014044657

Written by and for amazing cancer patients everywhere

TABLE OF CONTENTS

FOREWORD by Russ Messing
PREFACE by Nancy Novack

SURVIVING UNCERTAINTY

HOPE FLOATS

BEND, DON'T BREAK

CONNECTIONS

WHAT IS COURAGE?

CANCER'S GIFTS

FOREWORD

Russ Messing
Chair of Nancy's List

KEEPING HOPE ALIVE has turned into a nationwide community event, thanks to the work of Nancy Novack.

Ten years ago, when my dear friend Nancy told us about her cancer diagnosis, shock, then sadness, and then the incredibly rapid dawning that this could be the end for our lifelong friendship struck us like so many blows. What did we do? We did not wallow. We did not beat our breasts. We jumped in with both feet. We drove with Nancy to her doctors' appointments, and sat with her in silence, in grief, in hope, and in encouragement. We shared her fears. We walked beside our friend both figuratively and literally. Of course, it helped that Nancy is an indefatigable optimist, a doer, and a courageous woman.

I won't have hair? Oh well, I'll get the most outrageous and glamorous wig. In fact, I'll get a few.

People will be afraid to talk to me about this? Oh, well, I'll talk about it, I'll demystify it, I'll enlist people's support. I'll create a nonprofit to help people deal with the shock, the reality, the disbelief, and the terror of the diagnosis.

My psychology practice will be negatively affected? Don't even think about it. I have a story to tell of courage and resilience and coping. How can that not be helpful to others?

Nancy's can-do attitude, her ability to fight through her fears and doubts, the fatigue, the pain, the uncertainty—all were and are essential in her one-step-at-a-time triumphs.

This book is one of those triumphs. It is for and because of you.

PREFACE

My name is Nancy Novack.

Ten years ago, I was diagnosed with stage IV ovarian cancer. It had metastasized into my liver. In "cancer talk," everything is compared to a fruit. My ovary was the "size of a grapefruit." My liver was two times its appropriate size, more like a "small watermelon." I was too happily innocent about the cancer world and said two now-remarkable things: "Thank goodness, it is not appendicitis," and "What is stage V?"

I was always blessed with a magnificent "A Team." These lovely people held my hand and my heart throughout the challenging journey.

I always knew I would make it. But this was "seriousness" and ultimately I had to "be with" my attitude toward my own death—how I might act in its presence or how I might handle it when it didn't seem imminent to me, but truly appeared to be to others. I had twenty-one very aggressive chemo treatments mixed in with many complications. My attitude was always one of gratitude juxtaposed with enormous denial that I would be anything but very well again. Denial was my way of escaping sadness.

During my very long chemo sessions, whenever I had the

opportunity, I invited patients to tell me their stories. They shared feelings of helplessness and hopelessness. They worried about being present and honest with their children and not knowing what to say to them, about telling their employers and likely losing their jobs, about the potential for bankruptcy and foreclosure, about the loss of insurance or the inability to pay for their medications. They suffered feelings of isolation, fear, distrust, anger, and profound sadness.

I made a vow to make a difference for people living with cancer, for those who love and care for them, and, particularly, for the children who have a cancer diagnosis or love someone who has. My simple and profound wish is that *no one will ever go through cancer alone.* To bring purpose and meaning to my cancer path, I went deep into my heart to find new ways to help: by using my skills as a psychologist specializing in family systems, and by sharing the open hearts of my oncologist, my loved ones, and all those I have met and loved on this cancer path.

I created Nancy's List in the San Francisco Bay Area in 2008 as my "love letter" to the universe, an expression of my profound gratitude for my miraculous recovery and my life. Nancy's List is a community partnership to meet the epidemic of cancer. We know that we cannot rely on the healthcare system to focus on the many physical, psychosocial, and spiritual challenges that come with a cancer diagnosis. We *can* rely on our humanity. We *can* reach out and support the courage, bravery, and resilience of our neighbors.

At our first Love Fest, I said, "It takes a village to deal with the enormity of the cancer crisis in our community. I want to build one to do that." I placed clipboards around the party room in Sausalito asking for sign-ups—to drive their neighbors to treatments, to babysit their children, to walk the family dog, to prune the roses, to prepare and deliver healthy meals, and more.

Everyone got it!

Through our programs, cancer patients and their loved ones find community, strength, courage, healing relationships, and they laugh a lot. There is healing power when one is connected to the larger community, especially when you are experiencing fear, loneliness, isolation, and uncertainty. It means everything to know your neighbors are looking out for you, to share pleasurable experiences with your loved ones, to meet kindred spirits along the path. Cancer patients are truly moved by the many angels in our midst. It does take a village to handle this crisis, *and* we are building a magnificent one.

No one will ever go through cancer alone is the mission of Nancy's List and Nancy's Club (a club for children who have a cancer diagnosis and/or those who love someone who has). We want every man, woman, teenager, and child who has to walk the walk to hold the hand of someone who has been there, someone who understands the cancer mystery, and who can hang in there when times are tough.

For me, cancer changed everything. It generated my growth. It taught me the essence of gratitude, especially for the generosity of strangers. It refined my calling and defined my purpose as a psychologist. It gave me the opportunity to offer hope to those who have lost theirs.

I found courage and resilience.

And cancer opened my heart . . . to love again, to trust again, and to let myself be loved. It gave me permission to live and love with wild abandon.

Please accept *I Am with You* as an offering of friendship to sustain you on the first frightening nights after hearing a diagnosis, and every night thereafter. I am with you. As are all of the writers who have grappled with cancer themselves or alongside loved ones. *I Am with You* is a book of hope, wisdom, wit, inspiration, compassion, and love. It is so good, so rich in detail and deep in feeling.

Every story you read speaks to the power of those simple, exquisite words spoken to me by my dear oncologist Dr. Branimir Sikic, "I am with you."

SURVIVING UNCERTAINTY

"We are fragile, but we are also divine."
—*Cheryl Crow*

HOPE

Dagmar Herbstreuter

> *For all those who held my hand in the process,
> especially "My Simon" and Ingrid.*

The three little words that turned my world upside down came on March 13, 2013. They were not the "I love you" fairy tale happy ending kinda words, but the devastating diagnosis, "You have cancer."

Talk about a soul punch. Never having experienced such pain before, the only way I could describe it to my husband was that my soul hurt.

What I recall of those first days now is absolute craziness. After I was given my diagnosis, my first words were, "Can somebody please call my work and tell them I can't come tomorrow?" Allison, my little angel patient navigator, said these ever-wise words, "Dagmar, don't worry about it. *This* is your job now."

The week to come brought test after test, the horror and fear of awaiting results, and so many open questions. I was the poster child of good health—how was this possible?

So let your journey begin here:

Stop, it's done. For whatever reason or morbid lesson to be learned, you are the lucky number eight in the statistics. *But*, starting with the diagnosis, you are also a survivor.

So many times I had heard, "You will have to fight now," but

I didn't really know what that meant. How do you fight for your life? I very quickly realized that what I had to fight were two thoughts: why me? and poor me!

There is no point to these two agonizing thoughts.

Why me?, because getting cancer is random, you probably didn't do anything to get this.

Poor me, because it doesn't serve any purpose. Stop beating yourself up.

It will be a hard journey but you will find an amazing warrior within you.

You will lose your boobs.

You will most likely lose your hair.

There will be days that will be hard, really hard.

There will be days when everything sucks.

There will be days when you absolutely cannot get yourself together. Just accept it. As Elizabeth Gilbert says, "Embrace the glorious mess that you are." You don't have to be that strong, at least not every day. You can go into your cancer cave, just don't feel sorry for yourself.

It *will* pass.

I came to find that there is beauty at the core of the beast, and you will come out a stronger person than ever before. It's almost like magic. I had to accept and open myself to the outpouring of love and support. Because everyone I knew felt helpless, we were all carried on the same wave of love.

It is so very hard to give advice in this situation. Every story is different. Every person is different. You will find what works for you. We as human beings have amazing coping mechanisms.

Right away, we decided we didn't want to call my "condition" cancer. It's such an ugly word. So we decided to call it "crab." (Get it? The astrological sign for Cancer.) I had a crab card that I would pull without shame. Cancer has a wicked sense of humor. Find it.

Completely stressed out before my treatment started, I had an epiphany: I decided to let my brilliant doctors do their jobs, while I would do what was within my realm of possibilities and carry on my life as normally as possible.

I danced, I laughed, I cried. I found humor in cancer. I found a crazy sense of fashion. I found loads of love. I found incredible, strong, outrageous fellow survivors. Cancer patients are a special lot.

Life continues with all its craziness and tenderness and awesomeness and humor and heartbreak and love.

You can do it.

I wrap you in a big, warm hug—

Dagmar

WHAT HELPED ME THROUGH THE ANGST

My yoga practice has helped me greatly throughout my first phase of treatment. Sometimes, it was just sitting on the mat in my class, feeling connected and being part of a community.

P.S. Don't forget to talk to your "wig girl." She is an endless source of information!

GOT CANCER: *Now What?*

Paige Davis

There is really nothing that can prepare you for a cancer diagnosis. It is a shocking and momentary devastation that is overwhelming on so many different levels—physically, emotionally, and spiritually. But perhaps the greatest challenge is identifying the immediate logistical next steps of what a diagnosis means while you are trying to process these levels.

Below is a "best of the best" advice list, that I both learned through experience and received from others during those first few weeks of my cancer diagnosis. I have found these to be helpful to my personal journey (realizing that for everyone it is different).

1. *It's okay to freak out.*
Yes, this is a big deal. You could die.

2. *You probably won't die.*
Or at least you don't have enough information to know yet. Many cancers are very treatable, so honor the initial freak out and start arming yourself with some information to empower your journey.

3. *Find a team you trust.*
The number one recommendation that I wish someone had told

me was to meet with an oncologist first (versus a surgeon). An oncologist will talk you through the type of cancer you have and provide a recommendation of a treatment plan and ideally a recommendation of a surgeon he or she trusts. An oncologist is likely to provide more of a holistic and emotional understanding of the disease, whereas some surgeons (although not all) tend to be more straightforward and direct in their approach.

For my family and me, this direct approach from a surgeon as our first consultation was too shocking and harsh. In hindsight, perhaps it was simply because it was our first meeting and denial was met head on with reality. I ultimately ended up at MD Anderson with the same treatment plan as was prescribed by the first surgeon we met, but the approach was so much different.

Note: If you choose to go an alternative path, I still recommend hearing both sides of Western and Eastern approaches. I always thought that if I were to ever get cancer, I would go the alternative route. But as soon as I heard how treatable my breast cancer was and the science to support it, I chose the Western path but had a very comprehensive complementary approach alongside it (meditation, acupuncture, diet, exercise, etc.).

4. Get a second opinion.
This was the last thing I wanted to do, but my family really encouraged it. I just wanted to find my medical team and get the tumor out of me. It really is a good idea to get a second opinion—ideally from a cancer center of excellence. It's likely they will validate the initial recommendation you heard, but they could have an approach, insight, or other information that could be helpful. Ultimately, it is your decision.

5. This really is the worst time.

Or at least the most overwhelming time, with all the appointments, understanding insurance coverage, sharing with friends and family. Everyone told me that I would feel so much better when I had a plan in place. And they were right. I wasn't prepared for the plan taking up to three to six weeks to have in place. Assuming you don't need immediate surgery or treatment, have patience and know that you will feel some peace soon.

6. Suck it up and let people help.

Whether you choose to be very public in sharing your diagnosis, as I was, or private, people are going to want to help, and you are going to need it. For most of my life, I was convinced I could do everything on my own, so I saw this as my opportunity to let go and embrace the support surrounding me. As family and friends can attest, I got very good at asking for help and articulating my needs very quickly. (We are now working on boundaries.) Be specific and think about things that would be helpful (grocery runs, play dates for your kids, flowers, meal drop-off, etc.).

7. Stay off the Internet.

One of the best pieces of advice I received was to have a friend or family member do the online research for you. At the end of the day, you should be relying on your medical team to advise you, but it is too tempting not to get online. Having said that, there is some really f*#@ed up stuff out there, and this is the last thing you need to be dealing with. My mom became my online-research guru. Granted, at times I had to advise her to step away from the computer, but she really became the go-to source for distilling the information that would be helpful for me.

8. *Be prepared.*

I come from a very strategically minded family, so we were beyond prepared with key questions for each appointment. Contrary to the above advice to stay off the Internet, this is the time to get online with searches that are very specific (questions to ask my oncologist about breast cancer treatment). There are some great resources out there.

9. *Celebrate, or at least go to a silly movie.*

For me, it was important that I celebrate the milestones. Before my bilateral mastectomy, my friends threw me a "bye-bye boobs brunch." We had a "chemo kick-off" party the evening before chemo. While they were all important milestones, these events were more distractions that plucked me out of the intensity of the time with some good food, friends, family, and laughter.

10. *It's gonna be a rough year. But then it is over.*

This was perhaps the most important piece of insight I gained from several friends, that I am only now just coming to appreciate. I remember when my doctor told me it would be a year of surgeries and treatment, I was devastated. I could not even imagine a year of feeling this uncertain, sick, and scared. And they were all right. It was a really shitty year (the better I start to feel, the more I realize how difficult it was).

But now, as I am re-emerging on the other side with newness all around me (new hair, new perspective, new possibilities), I can see it as the most transformative and healing year of my life. I also realize how fortunate I am that it was just a year, which is not always the case. Sure, I will always be living in a post-cancer world, but for the most part, this phase is over.

And like these tips about handling your diagnosis, I am

realizing that the lessons learned over this past year are not so much about cancer as they are about life.

Originally appeared in *The Huffington Post*, 2014

MY HEALING GAME PLAN (WHICH I PRETTY MUCH STUCK TO)

My game plan for myself, my friends, and family —

Hello family. Hope everyone is doing well. Really appreciate the love and support over the last few days. It still seems surreal, and I know the next couple of weeks will likely be the most overwhelming with the influx of data that will be coming in. Knowing this, I have set up my alternative healing plan at a high level and articulated some initial guidelines I'd like to share with everyone.

I get that this is my way of coping for now, and assure you I have had my breakdown moments and am not naive to what lies ahead. But I also think that this is a crazy ironic gift, and I must be open to receiving whatever lessons I can, and I believe the plan below will help me and all of us to do this. Welcome to Team Woo!

Team Woo Alternative Plan
(for Paige — but you are welcome to partake)

EVERYDAY REGIME
• *Meditation — thirty minutes at least once but ideally twice a day*
• *Visualization — once a day on the actual mass, focusing on shrinking mass*
• *Energy Work — once a week/every two weeks*
• *Talk Therapy — once a week (one-on-one, group, etc. — all TBD)*

- *Flowers—fresh flowers, weekly*
- *Accessories—stones, oils, feng shui house cleaning, edibles, etc. (all TBD, based on need)*

COMPLEMENTARY REGIMEN
(to discuss with doctor, pending treatment plan)
- *Hypnotherapy*
- *Nutrition*
- *Reflexology*
- *Acupuncture*

Team Woo Guidelines
(recommended only—at the end of the day—your process)

1. This Is a Love Journey:
While shitty, it is happening. I prefer to stay away from terms about fight, battle, or referring to treatments as poison. It is all healing energy, and this is a love journey that the universe has invited each of us on. Not to say we can't have some attitude— after all, this cancer chose the wrong fucking body. My goal is to be as present as possible with each step and try not to get too far ahead of myself.

2. Reach Out for Support:
As we all know, this is often hardest on the caretakers. I hope everyone has embraced this. It is now as much a part of your journey as it is mine—I am just driving the bus. I need to know that everyone is taking care of herself or himself, but realize I need to let go and leave that up to each of you. Whatever feelings of fear, confusion, anger, resentment are coming up, please seek support—ideally outside the family. I will be planning on attending

many support groups, as well as a combination of traditional therapists. I'm not saying you should see a therapist, but I am sure there are support groups for families of cancer patients, and I encourage you to explore that (you get to be anonymous). Or, at a minimum, reach out to friends.

3. *Game Day Rituals:*
It is important to me, on the day of any meetings, treatments, or surgeries, that everyone be as grounded as possible. For you, it can be just taking a few deep breaths. I will be personally visualizing these experiences and sending light to the doctors, nurses, the office staff, etc. At whatever level this resonates, I want to invite them to be part of the Love Journey (whether they feel this or not). Also, it is important that everyone feels the best they can on these days. That can mean dressing super comfy, or it could mean dressing in full-on glamour. Whatever the case, please treat yourself with total self-love, empowerment, and compassion. I will also be carrying pods (a stuff 'n' go bag from BlueAvocado — the company I co-founded) at all times for those moments when I feel compelled to practice spontaneous gifting, and you should do the same.

4. *One Day at a Time:*
I am not naive; this will be a long journey. But I want to celebrate the milestone of each step, once we have an understanding of those steps. I am not sure what that looks like, but I believe this will be helpful in staying present to the process of healing.

I love you all so much and am sure more guidelines will be added, but this is what immediately has come to mind.

Love you all,
Paige

FORMING ATTACHMENTS, NEAR AND FAR

Susan Gubar

One of the most unforeseen benefits of living with cancer is the intimacy it creates with individuals we barely know. Affections spring up with surprising force.

About a succession of complaints, Virginia Woolf believed that "the best of these illnesses is that they loosen the earth about the roots. They make changes. People express their affections."

I considered Woolf's words when we were coming out of the Polar Vortex, much of which I spent hibernating, knitting a cowl with bulky wool on thick needles for the nurse who has helped me stay alive these past two years. Sage green was the color I had chosen for Alesha. Warm and bumpy in the seed stitch, the circular scarf would look gorgeous against her beautiful complexion.

Every time I see Alesha, she says, "You make everything too easy for me." As the research nurse of the clinical trial in which I am enrolled, she is the one who makes everything easier by scheduling the blood tests and CTs, distributing the pills, producing the diaries, reminding me where I have to be when, overseeing the taking of vitals, sending me test results, and recommending measures to alleviate the effects of treatment.

Although we reside sixty miles apart and will never visit each other's homes, if I am frightened or fraught by a fever or ache, I email her with confidence that she will advise me. I know next to nothing about Alesha's personal life, but I feel deeply grateful and connected to her.

Passionate attachments exist between cancer patients, too. A person I hardly knew now resides in my heart. A colleague a few years younger than I at another state university, she had produced scholarship I admired. But we had met only a few times before she confronted the cancer with which I struggle. Why should having the same disease bond people? Every week, I looked forward to our Sunday phone conversations about teaching and parenting and debilitating treatments.

After a recurrence and bouts of depression, my friend overcame her resistance and embarked on another cycle of chemotherapy. Yet at the start of April, she said on the phone: "I am divesting myself. I can't endure another miserable winter like this one." I was glad she had found a palliative care physician, but her decision to give away her scarves deeply unsettled me. No, it tore me up.

While I considered various yarns for a warm cowl she might enjoy wearing, I realized that, as with Alesha, I would probably never know the color of my friend's coat. Yet we closed our weekly phone conversations with heartfelt attestations of devotion. How strange that the evils of cancer beget the blessings of such ardor.

When I delivered the sage green stole to Alesha, she opened the recycled Macy's box and exclaimed, "Oh, it's an infinity scarf" as she looped it around her neck and then pulled up the back to make a hood.

Thinking of that conversation, of casting on as well as casting off, and of the coming fair weather, I went to my closet and chose a paisley silk sent decades ago by my collaborator and a lightweight pashmina brought to the hospital by a well-wisher. At my desk, I addressed a mailer and then found a card in which I wrote my message:

Darling, I am divesting myself of these scarves to invest them with you so you can divest and invest for us both. Love, Susan.

Only weeks later, when my friend's chemotherapy failed and she enlisted the aid of hospice, did I find the words that convey what I really had wanted to communicate. A "Prayer" by Galway Kinnell expresses, much better than I could, my aspiration for her and for myself.

> *Whatever happens. Whatever*
> *what is is is what*
> *I want. Only that. But that.*

Read these words aloud to yourselves and slowly, I would have implored my undergraduates (before doing so myself more than once, even as they rolled their eyes).

Kinnell, urging himself toward acceptance, encourages us to pause, to settle on all three iterations of the word "is." He wants to embrace existence, its joys and its miseries. The final phrase, tinged with stubborn defiance, asks at the very least for the recompense of hard-won assent. Admittedly, his mantra remains challenging for those of us living or dying with cancer and for those upon whom we depend. Yet I cherish the moments when it wraps me in changes.

Oh beloved friend: Though you were not given the time you needed, though I realize how bereft your husband and children and friends feel, I hope the transient peace these words instill in me finally enveloped you, as I now struggle to endure your absence from the world your presence graced.

But you, with your keen sense of injustice, might have wanted me to close by railing against the grievous losses inflicted by the detestable disease and inadequate treatments we decried together, and honoring your bright spirit, so I fervently do.

From *The New York Times*, 8/28/2014

TO MY NEXT THIRTY CANCER-FREE YEARS

Benjamin Rubenstein

A friend of mine did not want to celebrate her thirtieth birthday. She hadn't accomplished what she had expected. She drowned in a void—her hollowness filled with a ticking clock, save-the-date cards, movies and shows with typical American happy endings. To her, thirty was not part of the linear ascent but rather a cliff. "You can either feel young or wise," she said.

There are many things to count besides years of living. As a boy, I counted my baseball cards, specifically the ones with Ken Griffey, Jr., and Cal Ripken, Jr. I counted the minutes until I was allowed to finish practicing piano. I counted each passed week during summer break, glowing after only one and sulking with only a few left.

When I was sixteen and seventeen, I watched the hour-countdown on my IV pump, rejoiced at the beep, watched the next hour-countdown, and rejoiced at the next beep. I counted the drips of anti-tumor drugs. Some staggered, clumped together, and formed one large drip. Others followed one after the other. I counted down until bedtime so that I could begin again the next day.

I counted the days after cancer surgery until I could eat a Cinnabon and wear my favorite yellow Adidas pants. I counted the minutes until radiation sessions ended and days until I didn't need any more radiation.

When I was nineteen, with my second cancer, I counted the days until I found a bone marrow donor and both rejoiced and cowered when that countdown ended. After my transplant, I counted the days until I was allowed to step outside my hospital room to read the gossip magazines in the nook. I tallied my vomits and both rejoiced and felt disappointment when they stopped. I wanted to reach triple digits.

I counted the months until I weaned off immunosuppressants and the years until I completed my inoculations and reached my five-year cancer-free marks. I sometimes counted how much of my life was stolen by cancer, how far behind I was and how fast I'd have to catch up. I liked to think treatment slowed cell aging which allowed me to retain my youth, though more than likely my maturity just remained that of a teenager.

Then I counted the medications I stopped taking; the plummet in heartbeats per minute and increase in iron plates during exercise; the decrease in ferritin in my blood and increase in bone mineral density; the body fat I shed; the girls I went out with and the ones I was too scared to ask; the books I finished on Kindle. I estimated my calorie consumption for fat-burning, maintenance, and cheat days. The last estimate is the most challenging and fun.

And I counted the hundreds of thousands of dollars I would need before I could afford a home in Washington, DC; the days lost commuting; the video gaming, pranks, sleep, fun, travels, and adventures lost being a real adult. I counted the Washington Redskins' losses until I couldn't count any higher.

I think of my next traveling and rock-climbing adventures; the next new inspiring friend I'll meet; the next time I'll think I'm in love three minutes after meeting someone; the next task I'll help my parents with; the Samsung Galaxy S XXXIII; other uses for flying drones; my future fantasy football keeper players.

I think of how long I'll live if I keep getting allergy shots and eating cauliflower. Probably 150.

When I was a boy, I hated shrimp and now I could eat Bang Bang Shrimp at Bonefish Grill every day. Timelines and expectations we have set for ourselves can change, too, and like how a horizon changes based on the observer's position, one viewpoint is not lesser than the other.

I will embrace turning thirty this month and continuing to feel young and unwise—after all, I have 120 more years to learn.

Benjamin is the author of
Secrets of the Cancer-Slaying Super Man.
See more at *www.cancerslayerblog.com*

HOW IS THIS FOR WHAT MADE MY HEALING HAPPEN?

Junk food, fast food, milkshakes, double milkshakes, triple milkshakes; sports, Redskins, NFL Sundays, baseball playoffs, Derek Jeter; video games, friends coming over to play video games, skipping normal responsibilities to play video games; did I mention milkshakes?

A LITTLE WORSE FOR SOME WEAR

Max Jennings

These days when I'm driving and a song from the past few years comes on the radio, I hastily change the station, my fingers scrambling with the flimsy plastic presets. Even if I'm quick, the familiar words or melodies trigger what I've come to call "bad thoughts." No matter how positive recent tests have been, some things still trigger memories of the first nights after my diagnosis.

I found the first tumor on my testicle on the night of the 2013 Super Bowl. I was in the middle of my junior year at the University of Southern California. Earlier in the day, I'd finished a long training run, so initially I chalked the discomfort up to a pull in my groin. The pain certainly wasn't acute.

I went outside to the concrete slab my roommates and I called a backyard, and frantically felt at the hard spot on my right testicle. A quick Internet search found page after page assuring me there were other things it could be. But something just felt so wrong, I knew it was none of those things.

Two days later, the diagnosis was final.

Cancer.

The days between diagnosis and the start of treatment are the worst, at least for me. I would lie in bed at night, knowing there was something inside me that would kill me if left unchecked, and it was unchecked.

Two surgeries and a few months of recovery later, I was back in Los Angeles for school. At the time, I remember telling people that three months of interruption wasn't a lot in what would presumably be a long life. I'm sure that would have held true, but last fall, the cancer came back.

I got the call from my doctor a few minutes before I had intended to leave for the grocery store. I always shopped on Wednesday nights, because the store wasn't busy. Instead of calling my parents, I went to the store anyway.

Getting into the car, I turned the radio up as loud as the built-in speakers of a 2003 Toyota Matrix would go. The music rattled the windows. It felt good. For a moment, the music enveloped everything, and I didn't feel scared or tired.

Under the harsh fluorescent lights of the beer aisle, I studied the selection and picked an expensive brand from San Francisco.

The cashier bent my flimsy Minnesota ID between his fingers and paged the manager.

"You can just walk away, buddy," he said, sneering like he enjoyed accusing students of using fake IDs.

"It's not fake. Why would I use a fake that made me look younger?"

"We'll see, buddy."

"My cancer came back today, so maybe we could just skip this part?"

Improbably, the line worked.

I had three strong beers and watched music videos with a roommate I hadn't told yet.

"Blood tests will catch a return of the disease before you feel it," I had been told.

So I'd ignored the building sense of wrong for a few weeks and not gone in to see the doctor, until one of the tumors was visibly bulging out of my neck.

Chemo started the day after my twenty-second birthday. "The night before chemo" is the worst birthday party theme ever, if anyone is wondering.

A lot of things have been said about the contradictions of a process which injects chemicals so toxic the nurses sometimes wear hazmat suits, but it kept me alive, so I have to be grateful, however tough the process was.

Once chemo was over, I was right back to waiting. Waiting for tests that would confirm if the chemo had worked, waiting to get a regular life back.

My trust in my body has come to depend on how recently I've had tests. It grows progressively weaker the further I get from the reassurance of an encouraging test result.

The physical part of fighting cancer is hard, but the mental fight is much harder. Well, maybe not harder, but far less straightforward. I try to focus on a future when I'm healthy and treatment has been effective. Most of the time this works, until suddenly it doesn't, and I'm in bed trying to sleep and all I can think about is the ache in my neck.

There is always a chance the disease will return, that the next round of treatment won't work. In these moments, I feel like I'm living with a clock that is accelerating toward the end. I can practically hear the ghostly ticks in my quiet bedroom.

But there's a clock on everyone's life. I just have a specific place to focus my worries.

I've realized I need to enjoy the world to the best of my ability. Especially with the people who have made my life so rich that the thought of it ending prematurely is so gut-wrenching. These are the people who've cooked meals, sent gifts, made mix tapes, or just sat and been sad with me for a moment.

They have offered words of fear, struggle, and bittersweet memory. Yet these are almost always matched by expressions of hope, love, and pure curiosity about the world, and ways we can make it a better place. Many stories of family and friends come and gone have been offered. These people may be out of sight at the moment, but they are etched deeply into our collective hearts.

I often fantasize about running away and starting over without all this baggage, but then I remember the scars the disease has left on my body and mind. They will not just disappear with a new place and new people.

But they will fade with time.

I love so much around me with all of the pieces of my shattered heart. Some things cannot be put back together, but I'm not one of them.

This is meant to tell of the trauma of surgeries, multiple diagnoses, and chemo. I want people who have to go through something similar to know that it is hell, that by the time it is over you will be different. There will be wear on your body and mind, but that doesn't mean that you will be sadder. There will be struggles with anxiety and maybe even depression, but there are people who can help. If anything, after two years of constant struggle to stay alive, I'm probably happier than I was before. I have friends, family, and communities who have supported me through so much. People here and there have remarked that a period of struggle can make you wiser. At this point, I often feel like it just makes clear how much I don't know. I am just hopeful I get a full life to try to figure a tiny fraction of it out.

The process has been longer and harder than I thought it would be, but I think I will make it.

Just maybe, a little worse for some wear.

Originally appeared in *Reimagine.me*, 2014

I'M GLAD I HAD . . .

1. A golden retriever. Or two, as it happened.

2. Favorite foods. I have heard people say not to eat your favorite foods during chemo, but I did, and I still like them, and it made me happy.

3. Lots of hats. I asked for hats on Facebook and was sent about seventy from all over the world. Do specify that they not all be knitted because scratchy wool was hard on my scalp after the hair fell out.

4. Blankets, and warm clothing, if you live in a cold climate. I did chemo from December to February in Minnesota.

5. TV. I had delusions that I would be productive during chemo. Nope. Just watch TV, enjoy what you can, and get through it.

THE ART OF FALLING

Steven Baum

I know how to fall. I realized this in midair.

After a year of training for a triathlon, and just days before the race, I crashed my bike at 40 mph into the side of a crossing pickup truck. Doctors and nurses were all shocked that I survived. They repeatedly told me I should be dead, or at least severely paralyzed. Not only did I survive, I escaped without head, neck, or spinal injuries, or even road rash. Surprising to me, I knew how to fall and it saved my life.

I now realize that knowing how to fall is less about physical talent and more about mental acceptance. It's about embracing the reality of the moment. In the few seconds before I hit the truck, when it was clear that I was going to crash, I unexpectedly let go. Thankfully, this was an uncharacteristic moment. For once in my life, I did not try to control the situation. I did not try to cleverly maneuver the bike. I did not even brace myself. I was without tightness or resistance. The bike took the full impact of the collision; I was launched over the hood of the truck, landing face down on the asphalt. Four broken bones in my pelvis. Alive.

I imagine that being diagnosed with cancer is like crashing into that truck. Everything is fine, until that instant when it isn't. Life becomes barely recognizable. The flood of unanswerable questions quickly starts to come. *Will I live? For how much longer? Am I strong and brave enough to survive? Will I suffer? Will it be painful? Will I die? Will I make the right choices? Will family and friends support me? Do I have the best medical care? Will I tolerate and respond to treatment?* And the anxious noise goes on, and on, and on.

This was the case for my sixty-year-old mother, Nancy Novack, who, after complaining about abdominal pain to her internist, was diagnosed with stage IV ovarian cancer. A virtual death sentence, she miraculously beat it, defying overwhelming odds. More than ten years have now passed, and doctors are still mystified by her ability to overcome such dire circumstances.

Many say that surviving cancer is all about the fight. Watching my mother go through her diagnosis, aggressive treatment, and eventual recovery convinced me that, paradoxically, it's actually about letting go. Just like in those fleeting seconds before I hit the truck, she embraced her situation with a rare and enviable calmness. And, like me on the bike, I think she surprised herself with a newfound grace and resolve. She didn't resist cancer, or try to control it. She ignored the noise, aware that so much was out of her control. She focused on her desire to live today, knowing that this was all she could control and all that mattered.

My mother mastered the art of falling, and it saved her life.

"I AM WITH YOU"

Nancy Novack

My decision to create this anthology came from my fascination with and curiosity about what makes one patient get well, despite the diagnosis, and another, despite the diagnosis, perish. And what roles do hope and despair bring to these outcomes? How does one prepare one's self to face the challenges and the traumas of cancer treatment? I want to eradicate the wicked disease, and I am passionate about that. I am truly fortunate to have outlived my cancer diagnosis. I want to use myself and my experience to bring a sense of hope, a sense of belonging to a greater community, to encourage my sisters and my brothers to receive the blessings of those who have walked the cancer walk before. That is the spirit in which this anthology was conceived.

On April 29, 2004, I was diagnosed with stage IV ovarian cancer which had metastasized to my liver. I had no idea what any of that meant, despite living on this planet, mostly in northern California, for sixty years. I didn't know anything about the treatment, the statistics, what was ahead of me. And I had no one to journey with me who had survived the same diagnosis.

It didn't take long to get it. As is true of any teaching hospital, Stanford is notorious for sending out the troops to inspect every square inch of the body of an "interesting" case. That's what they do, and they come in droves, and they ask a million questions, and they probe away.

The severity of the situation started to hit me, although it was still so very surreal. The surgeons came, sharpening their scalpels, ready to go. My sweet cousin Leslie tried to manage the many terribly serious conversations on that first momentous day, all the while holding my hand and my heart. She really managed everything, and beautifully.

I am in a lovely room at Stanford Cancer Center gazing onto the flower gardens, feeling in an altered state of no-consciousness, as if I were watching someone else's movie. After several hours of the procession of medical staff—professors, fellows, assistants, nurses, and the curious bystanders—a man walks into my room, looking a bit like Santa Claus. My recollection is that I say to him, "And who might you be?" and he announces he is my *doctor*. There is silence, a powerful sensitivity as we look right into the other's eyes. The healing begins.

What really healed me? My relationship with Dr. Branimir Sikic, his courage, caring, intelligence, and unwavering commitment to get me well from that very first night. He announced to the bevy of eager surgeons impatiently waiting in the corner, "Nancy has no time for surgery. We will start treatment and chemo immediately." There was tension in the room, the sense that the physicians who live by the FDA protocol might be in for some surprises.

He told me, "Yours is a very bleak diagnosis. It will be a rocky road. But hang in there. I think I can help you. I am with you." In those words, Brandy showed profound compassion. The kind of hope—the kind of love—that he exhibited throughout my treatment define the essence of this man.

He looked around the room, crowded with my friends and loved ones, and said, "When all those who love you go home tonight and you start to freak out about what has happened today, here is my home phone number. Feel free to call me." And I did, at about 2:30 in the morning. And Brandy was as gracious and generous in that phone call as he has always been, ever since.

Brandy Sikic really held my hand and my heart. Our relationship is based on trust. The deal we made was pretty simple: if ever something in my body felt different or wrong, my job was to contact him immediately. And he responded immediately from wherever he might be in the world. He never dismissed my calls or my fears and, rather, guided me through the next step—an emergency CT scan at midnight at Stanford, an emergency visit to Sloan-Kettering when my arm wouldn't move. Even when Brandy was on sabbatical in his hometown in Croatia, he was within earshot (email and phone call), and he made the critical decisions about my treatments. When the oncology team was considering a liver transplant, he weighed in daily with his directives. Again, no surgery because of Brandy. We did not do the transplant. And all is well.

Few doctors have said to their patients what Brandy once said to me, but I wish they would. "This is very tough. I am giving you very aggressive treatments. If you are on antidepressants, double them. If you are not on them, get on them. And find yourself a solid psychologist, preferably someone who has been through cancer."

Brandy made it possible for me to really trust—in him, the entire medical team, and the world. I was told that I could not do a lot of alternative methods while I was in treatment, since I was being so closely monitored. When my sweet sister asked if I could have ice cream, Brandy said, "This is not the time to deprive Nancy of any pleasures."

With this and so many other instances of extraordinary kindness and understanding over the past ten years (he brought me nine of his home-grown garden roses to celebrate my ninth anniversary from the date of diagnosis), Dr. Sikic laid the foundation within my spirit for true trust: an opening of my heart to the amazing generosity of strangers, to the compassion and sensitivity of the chemo infusion teams, to other patients, and to the beauty of my friends and loved ones. When people ask, and they often do, *What happened? How did you make it when others did not?* I don't have any answers to that mystery. I do know, for certain, that the opening of my heart, the receiving of the blessings and the love, the sense of abundance of good will coming my way changed my being—during my cancer and forever more.

Those four words, *I am with you,* are my four favorite words in the world. They sustained me, gave me hope, and transformed my understanding of the healing process. Every story in this anthology speaks to the power of those simple, exquisite words.

I am the luckiest lady in the world. I truly enjoy defying medical statistics and being the poster child for Stanford's Cancer Center.

I am immensely grateful.

WHAT HELPED ME THROUGH THE NIGHT

My A Team. And tons of sweetheart family and friends, who came from my kindergarten classes to now, and many people I never had the honor of knowing before my diagnosis. Of course, my then-dogs Fanny and Alexander, my still-African grey parrot Floyd.

Doing magic tricks with Russ with our plan to "take it on the road," horseback riding at Miwok Stables, yoga, many cool wigs, silk pajamas, painting my house periwinkle blue (my healing color), and falling in love.

I took several workshops with Dr. Rachel Naomi Remen, which were directed to psychologists for continuing education training. Upon arriving in my white furry boots, sharing a twinkle with very twinkly Rachel, I realized my purpose in being there was to define and refine my personal relationship to my cancer. I do recall that I did the same workshop three years in a row . . . . I really wanted to go deep into understanding my path.

One of the very powerful gifts that Rachel gave to me was an exercise called Keeping a Heart Journal. To quote Rachel,

"Most of us live far more meaningful lives than we know. Meaning is a function of the heart, an organ of vision that allows us to see below the surface of things. . . . Our habitual way of seeing things and even our expertise can blind us to the meaning of even the simplest of our daily interactions and relationships. Meaning is the antecedent of enduring satisfaction and fulfillment. . . . This simple little journal may be all that it takes to give us fresh eyes.

"Keeping a Heart Journal draws on the wise work of Angeles Arrien, author of The Fourfold Way. *This exercise requires a*

notebook to write in and ten to fifteen minutes of time every day. It is best to do this exercise at the same time and place—every evening if possible—and to find a quiet place to reflect and write where you will not be interrupted.

"Begin by sitting in silence for a few minutes and paying attention to your own breathing. At the end of each out-breath, there is a very brief moment of rest and peace before your next in-breath begins. See if you can notice this tiny natural space of stillness. Pay attention to it. Each time you arrive there, let yourself be there and surrender into the stillness as fully as you can.

"When you feel ready, begin the exercise by slowly reviewing your day backwards, going from the present moment back to the time when you awoke in the morning, recalling the events and conversations you experienced and the people you met as you moved through your day. Review your day backwards three times, each time asking yourself a different question.

"The first time you review your day backwards, ask yourself the question: 'What surprised me today?'

"As soon as you find anything that is an answer to this question, stop your review and write it down in your journal. It is not necessary to write a great deal or to find the most surprising thing that happened all day—the important thing is to re-examine your day from this new perspective and not how much you write about it.

"Now begin a review of your day once again, going from the present moment back to the time that you awoke in the morning, recalling the events and conversations you experienced, and the people you met.

"The second time you review your day backwards, ask yourself the question: 'What moved me or touched my heart today?'

"As soon as you find anything that is an answer to this question, stop your review and write it down in your journal.

"Now begin to review your day backwards a third time, going from the present moment back to the time that you awoke in the morning, recalling the events and conversations you experienced, and the people you met.

"The third time you review your day backwards ask yourself the question: 'What inspired me today?'

"As soon as you find anything that is an answer to this question, stop your review and write it down in your journal.

"This finishes the task for the day.

"Put your journal away until tomorrow. As time goes by, re-read your journal to yourself.

"Often when people first start this journal, they find the same answer to all three questions: 'Nothing. Nothing. And Nothing.' Do not be discouraged if this happens to you. Meaning is an innate capacity but also an acquired skill. If you do this exercise daily, before long, answers to all three questions will come to you.

"Sometimes you may notice that you were not surprised, touched, or inspired as you lived through your day, but that you are only surprised, touched, and inspired as you reflect and do this exercise. Do not be discouraged! Most people experience this time lag at first. After a while, you will begin to grow in your capacity to find that more and more things surprise, touch, and inspire you at the time they actually occur during the day. When this happens, notice any change in your attitude towards your life and those around you."

Applications:

"This exercise has many creative applications. You may want to set up this exercise process with your support group. Sharing parts of your journals will give everyone a far deeper appreciation of each other and of the rich nature of your shared experience. Children as young as eight are able to do this exercise and many enjoy it immensely. Doing this exercise with your family and sharing what has been written once a week can have surprising results—revealing the inner life of the family and the many ways we matter to one another without knowing."

I have done this exercise so often right before I go to sleep and felt so appreciative. I have suggested it to many of my friends and therapy clients who are living with cancer. It works!

Thank you, dear Rachel, for so many things . . .

From her website Rachel Remen
www.rachelremen.com/keeping-a-heart-journal/

HOPE
FLOATS

"When you are alone with your soul,
that's what you have to decide,
are you willing to hang on to hope?"
—Allison W. Gryphon

WHERE THE WILD THINGS ARE

John Smith

> *"All the soarings of my mind begin in my blood."*
> *— Rainer Maria Rilke*

The seasons fold into one another like origami. Several days of hard frost caused my tomatoes to droop with dismay. As if on cue, east winds set the maples ablaze with fall color. Then a front of marine air, spring-like, collided with the desert breezes and snow dusted the valley.

My appreciation for the beauty of the natural world is tempered by my health. I have a blood cancer, multiple myeloma. The disease environment in which I now live comes with complications. In the last five years, I received treatments aimed at reducing the damage caused by this incurable malignancy. The cancer markers remain stable following extraordinary chemotherapy and an autologous stem cell transplant. I continue to take low dose oral chemo and steroids. I am healthy.

Nonetheless, in the wan light of this reality, I and the other wildlife still have autumn rituals to complete. Squirrels scamper along the fringe of the forest. Their cheeks bulge with food for winter. I pull cartloads of dead plants from my gardens while grosbeaks mob the elderberry. Other small birds twitter as they feast on the gone-to-seed flowers. I drain and roll my irrigation hoses; then I board up the crawl space beneath the house.

Toiling in one of my garden plots, I unearth remnants of my boys' imaginative childhoods. Toy soldiers and metal cars routinely appear when I work this piece of ground. Years ago, I'd dug a hole and filled the area with pavers' sand, atop which I built a small shelter. A ladder led to an eight-foot high platform. It was topped with a sheet metal roof that clattered in the Oregon rain. A thick-knotted rope hung from the roof beam and descended through a hole in the floor to the sandbox below. Here, my sons played until adventures on their bikes led them far from their home and innocence.

Against this backdrop of domestic familiarity and memories, I ponder on the finiteness of life. Everyone with cancer peers into the unknown of mortality, much like a child looks frighteningly into the world of adults. The territory of my contemplation is as magical as any child's daydream. It's scary . . . and thrilling. There are monsters with horns and big teeth. They howl and bark. A terminal illness steals from us the comfortable blanket of adulthood. We can no longer stroke its silky border of oblivion for security. Suddenly, we are awkward and self-conscious as adolescents; our hair falls out, our GI tract turns somersaults, or worse, freezes solid. Our body is not to be trusted. We sulk and just want to be alone.

Perhaps now is the time to consider the mischief we've made along the way. Probably, it's not as bad as we thought or others made us feel. Magic awaits; the world remains ours to behold. Cancer cannot foreclose on my astonishment at the mystery of life. For me, the wonder of being also glows in the terrible murky haunts of our perishability. At times, I am afraid; yet, I am nourished, encouraged even, by my fear. And, in the face of it, I'll continue to plan for the future.

My brain percolates with ideas for next spring's gardens. I envision more of one color here or there, maybe even a pond for the birds. It's nothing dramatic, just a few improvements to satisfy my imagination's appetite. The sandbox now belongs to me. I want to play there and, as for the monsters, well, they can join me. Together, we'll raise a rumpus.

Originally appeared in his website Good Blood, Bad Blood
www.goodbloodbadblood.wordpress.com

THE SIMPLE THINGS WORK FOR ME

It's always simple things with me. Initially, writing, walking, and my cats gave me comfort. To these meaningful activities, I recently added my first grandchild. She lights up my life.

LUBRICATE WITH LAUGHTER
Annie Sprinkle

I found laughter to be a great lubricant for getting through any tough times. My partner and I dressed up in silly costumes for chemo sessions. We made jokes about everything, as much as possible. Who said cancer can't be fun, silly, even hilarious?

Don't take it too seriously all the time. Yes, there are serious moments. But there are plenty of opportunities to play within the experience. I am here to say that I had fun with my breast cancer experience. But then, I had the luxury of early stage cancer. I don't know how I would have coped if it were later stage.

When you can, if you can, lubricate with laughter.

THE GRASS GROWS ALL BY ITSELF

Dr. Jerome Freedman

On Super Bowl Sunday, 1997, I went in for tests, a CT scan, and a cytoscopy, all of which led to a diagnosis of bladder cancer. From then to the next Super Bowl, and seventeen Super Bowls thereafter, I used every mindfulness and holistic practice I could to help with my path to healing.

One particular guided imagery session stands out. Two months after my diagnosis, I visualized myself with my wife at the top of a grassy hill, on our way down from a walk. Just then, I remembered a famous Zen poem:

Sitting quietly
Doing nothing
Spring comes
And the grass grows all by itself.

This poem came vividly into my mind. I realized that not only was I on the right path, but it was all downhill from here! I was filled with a feeling of tremendous bliss, which I harnessed into sending the positive energy directly into my bladder.

Then, the following poem popped into my mind, which I spoke out loud:

Lying still
Breathing in, breathing out,
Healthy cells grow all by themselves
I am free of cancer.

These became the watchwords of my healing experience. I used them to survive times of fear and darkness. I used them in the twelve years when I was cancer free. I used them again when the cancer returned in 2013. I even practiced them while walking, by repeating "healthy" as I placed my left foot down, and "free" as I placed my right foot down. Healthy and free. Free and healthy.

Through the long-enduring chemo side effects, through low blood counts and high creatinine test results, and through three afternoons of tennis at the club, I maintain this surprising practice. Healthy. Free.

I am on the path to a complete recovery from bladder cancer, where the grass—miraculously—grows all by itself.

WHAT NOURISHED ME
AND MADE MY HEALING HAPPEN

I am happy and grateful for the love and support of my family and friends through both episodes of muscle-invasive bladder cancer. Without them, I may have lost the belief that I could be made well again.

I am happy and grateful for the guidance and teachings of Zen Master Thich Nhat Hanh and the mindfulness practices that kept my mind in the present moment instead of worrying about the past and anticipating the future outcomes of my tests and surgeries.

I am happy and grateful for the care and advice I received from Michael Broffman and Dr. Marty Rossman about how to evaluate and combine the best of Eastern and Western medical treatments and supplement recommendations that supported my recovery.

I am happy and grateful for the skills I have developed in using the Internet to investigate the nature of bladder cancer and to present the probable diagnosis to my doctor before he gave it to me in 1997.

I am happy and grateful for the support groups I attended, such as the Center for Attitudinal Healing and Anna Halprin's dance and creative art cancer group, for guiding me into mental and emotional states that counteracted times of despair.

I am happy and grateful for the many guided imagery sessions I had with Leslie Davenport that brought out my internal resources for visualizing a complete response to all treatments.

I am happy and grateful for the opportunity to serve on the Board of Directors of the Marin AIDS Project and the Advisory Committee of the Institute for Health and Healing in order to give back to my community.

I am happy and grateful for being able to use the Pine Street Clinic for our Mindfulness in Healing well-being support and meditation group, and to meet there weekly since 2009.

A HEALTHY SPIRIT

Aenea M. Keyes

After hearing the shocking words, "You have cancer," how do you move forward? I heard the frightening words of that diagnosis twice, in 1997 and again in 2009. My journey back to health has taken me two decades. So I want to say that your journey to self-knowledge and self-love makes you a miracle . . . and a healthy spirit is what you are now creating.

In 1995, I learned that I had a rare form of kidney failure. Then, to complicate matters, I received an additional breast cancer diagnosis in 1997. This meant I had to wait to receive a kidney transplant. You have to be cancer free to get a transplant.

I had a mastectomy, and since my husband was not a match as a donor (and another family member—although a match— could not donate), I continued to wait for a kidney. Incredibly, within weeks of needing dialysis, an amazing friend volunteered to be my kidney donor in 2005! Both of my diseased kidneys were removed and the transplant was a success. Which made my bladder cancer diagnosis in 2009 an even bigger shock.

After unsuccessful chemo, a surgeon removed my bladder and replaced it, and then a long, slow recovery followed that was more challenging than the previous surgeries. I learned that courage, in this context, does not feel at all heroic, but more like an act of survival. Resilience also became a necessity. My inner strength, although usually in high reserve, was sorely tested. Painful life experience, if thought of as presenting an opportunity, becomes rich compost for the soul. I certainly got a complete life overhaul before I fully recovered.

You might ask how I kept my spirits up with all of these challenges. My husband and close friends, including my living donor, allowed me to feel the weight of my illness by witnessing my life and holding for me an emotional space of safety. The wonderful doctors, nurses, and other professional people who cared for me gave me hope with their genuine kindness and empathy, without feeling sorry for me. And at my husband's urging, my father reconnected with me after a decade's estrangement, and our shattered family began to heal.

Looking back, I now realize how fortunate I was that so many people offered their encouragement and wisdom. My breast cancer diagnosis included a short visit with a therapist. When this woman heard that I was thirty-two years old, and that my mother had died of cancer at age fifty, she amazed me. She said, "Your cancer is not your mother's cancer. Your outcome will be different and this is why . . ." Realizing that I would survive the breast cancer diagnosis was so empowering. A year later, I had a mastectomy of one breast. The cancer has not returned.

This may sound surprising, but it felt overwhelming adjusting to good health again, and fully reentering my life. I had lived with illness for so long. But my transplant physician reminded me that it is vital to stay focused on my particular path of health and fulfillment, no matter what others might think or say. Next year, I hope to mark the fifth anniversary of good health after my successful neobladder surgery.

Another supporter, a breast cancer nurse, said words that I will never forget: "When was the last time you felt joy? If you can't remember, you need to find joy right now, and try to feel it at least once a day!"

As a healthy spirit, I now know that once a day is not enough. Instead of thinking of joy as linked solely to happy feelings, I now know joy is within reach through living fully, feeling deeply, and taking pleasure in just simply being alive.

I am now heading for age fifty with a whole new optimism, thanks to the wisdom that so many have shared.

Please know that you—exactly as you are right now—are a miracle. As time goes on, you'll learn to see:

who can hear the truth of how you are feeling

who in your circle of family and friends loves you for who you are

who is comfortable with hearing about the details of your treatment

who can't hang in . . . and are best to be lovingly let go.

But most of all, you will learn to trust yourself, and to truly feel joy in the love of those who care about the one-and-only miraculous spirit—you!

WHAT MADE HEALING HAPPEN

Dark chocolate, my favorite comfy PJs, walks and talks with loved ones, nourishing food, comedy and mystery DVDs . . . embracing every kind of change . . .and fulfilling some dreams.

Enormous gratitude got me involved in this writing project—

to Nancy, your generosity embraces every cancer patient and survivor that crosses your path

to the many wonderful people who offered me their wisdom and compassion throughout my illness and recovery

to loved ones who continue to be at the heart of my support system—I am still here, because of you!

COPING WITH CANCER

Elana Rosenbaum

In the middle of a professional training session where I was teaching mindfulness-based stress reduction to healthcare professionals, I received a phone call from my husband. He wanted to give me the results of a biopsy on a lump in my neck. I wasn't too concerned about the test, as I felt well and stayed fit. I was surprised to learn I had Hodgkin's lymphoma.

As a psychotherapist and mindfulness teacher, it was my job to help people cope with troubling emotions and medical problems. Now I had to be, as I told others, "more than my disease" and focus on what was right rather than wrong with me. I knew that mindfulness, the ability to be in the present moment with clarity and kindness, would help me, as it has aided the thousands of patients I have worked with since 1984.

During treatment and throughout my recovery, I always carried a notebook and colored pencils to express in words and pictures feelings that could not otherwise be released. I promised myself not to suffer and to be open to all of my experiences, good and bad. Each moment became an opportunity to ride the waves of my thoughts, feelings, and sensations, and to find the place inside of me that was calm.

I discovered that not only had my body changed, but also my perceptions. Today, being aware of my mortality helps me stay alert. I do my best to resolve conflicts as they arise. I know the preciousness of relationships, love, and meaningful work. I try to be more kind and forgiving both to others and to myself. I recognize how easy it is to fall into negativity or burden myself with unrealistic expectations. My motto used to be: "It can always be worse." Now, it is: "Yes to life," and "Go for it."

Here at Dana-Farber, where I am now a patient, I was fortunate to teach meditation to patients, families, and staff at drop-in sessions and classes that highlight coping with cancer through mindfulness. My use of meditation while I had my stem cell transplant helped inspire a research study about how this approach can help staff.

During my recovery, I wrote a credo. Every now and then, I take it out and look at it. It says:

I resolve to dwell in the present and not be captured by fear. I shall use my experience to remember the preciousness of life and the gifts I have received. I shall challenge myself to live wisely and make meaning of my experience, letting it transform me. I shall work to bring peace to others, so they too may be free. I am filled with gratitude to all who have helped me be alive and well. May I never forget the grace that has been bestowed upon me.

It is not important what will be tomorrow. It is important to live today in harmony with myself and others and use the love I receive to give it out again. I shall work to maintain a balance, opening up to what is true, and acting accordingly. I shall not be ashamed of praise, but value my efforts, appreciate my bravery, and celebrate my joy. May I be able to: enjoy, replenish, dance, and sing; make love; care fully for my body and the spirit, and help others do the same.

May we all be well, and may I live with ease and happiness.

Originally appeared in *Mindful* magazine

THE PERMISSION SLIP

Allison W. Gryphon

Cancer sucks. There is no way around it, but I don't need to tell you that, you know. I will say that beyond the downside, cancer can bring many surprising good things into your life. Everyone is different. You will decide. That's the rule as far as I'm concerned. That you can fight cancer any way that you'd like.

Think of this as a blanket permission slip to be mad, sad, scared, happy, empowered, confused, exhausted, up, down, furious, and doubtful, but, most of all, use this as your permission slip to be hopeful.

Permission in place, my unsolicited encouragement is to be proactive and informed in all of your decisions and to remember that they are your decisions.

For me, stepping into the world of my cancer was stepping into a world of complete truth and authenticity. It allowed me to see on a profound level who I am and what I am made of. It gave me the opportunity to understand what was important for me in life, who was important, how I wanted to live, and what I wanted out of this world, all with no apologies. In a word, my cancer experience was liberating. Don't get me wrong, it was also a fight. I kept my focus on reaching the best outcome.

Do what feels right on your terms. Keep your eye on the prize. And go kick cancer's ass!

BEND, DON'T BREAK

"Cancer didn't bring me to my knees.
It brought me to my feet."
—Michael Douglas

TWO TINY GREEN BLADES OF GRASS:
The Will to Live

Rachel Naomi Remen

I am deeply honored to be asked to contribute some thoughts to this book. In thinking of what I have learned—after fifty-two years of practicing medicine and sixty-one years of personal experience with significant chronic illness—that might be useful to someone newly diagnosed, many things came to mind. There are countless articles and even books about them all. So I am writing about something closer and more personal, something woven into our very fabric that we may never have noticed; something that has made all the difference. Over time it has been called many names, but I would like to call it by one of the oldest: the Will to Live.

I first encountered the Will to Live as a young teen. I was walking up Fifth Avenue on a Saturday morning, window-shopping with my posse of friends, when a flash of green caught my eye. There, growing through the New York sidewalk, were two tiny green blades of grass. Small and tender, they had broken right through the cement to reach the sun. The image is still perfectly clear in my mind. As a New Yorker, I had never witnessed the power of living things before. I had been awed by the miracle of it.

My first personal experience with the Will to Live happened

several years later when I was a young physician. In 1981, I developed peritonitis and sepsis, when the sutures holding my intestines together gave way a few days after a six-hour abdominal surgery. By the time this was correctly diagnosed, I had become gravely ill. I was rushed back to the operating room where further surgery probably saved my life. I remember being pushed down a corridor at a dead run, the lights overhead flashing by, my surgeon, who was also my friend, running alongside my gurney. Medical culture being what it is, he was talking to me about my case as if we were two physicians lunching together in the doctors' dining room talking about a mutual patient. "You know," he said conversationally, "because of the infection, we will have to close by secondary intention." Filled with drugs and very ill, I remember thinking, "Secondary intention. I used to know what that means." Then events accelerated, and I lost track of it all.

Hours later, I awoke in the recovery room giddy with the realization that I had survived. Half conscious, I cautiously explored my abdomen with a fingertip. There was the same big soft bandage that had been there after each of my other surgeries. Comforted by the familiar, I drifted off.

The next morning, a nurse appeared to change my dressings. Chatting comfortably with me, she pulled back my bandages, and I looked down expecting to see the usual sixteen-inch incision with its neat row of a hundred or more stitches. Instead, there was a great gaping wound, as open as any I'd ever seen while assisting in the operating room. My surgeon's words came back to me in a rush—secondary intention—but today, I could remember what this meant. In the presence of infection, there could be no sutures. The surgical incision would simply be left open to heal on its own.

Deeply shocked, I looked down at the ruin of my abdomen. I remember thinking, "Surely this is a mortal wound. There is no way this can heal." My nurse chatted on cheerfully as she replaced my bandages, unaware of my shock. The next morning, she was back to change my dressing again. This time, I turned my face aside and closed my eyes. She spoke to me pleasantly as she tended to my physical needs. I didn't answer. I was in despair.

For several mornings, we went through this same routine together, she removing my bandages, murmuring encouragement, I, head averted, awaiting the end. After a week or so, it occurred to me that against all probability, I was still here. Perhaps I would not die of this great wound after all, but would have to live with it. This raised a completely different set of concerns and worries. How would I live with this great deep hole in my front? Perhaps, after many years, it might fill in and become flat, a scar sixteen inches long and several inches wide. In the meantime, how would I bathe? Could I wear extra large clothes or fill the deep trench in my belly with cotton so it would not show?

After a few days of such musings, it became obvious that if I were going to live with this, I would need to see it. So that day, when my nurse pulled back my bandages, I forced myself to look, expecting to see the huge gaping wound of ten days before. But it had changed. Astounded, I saw that it had begun closing in at the bottom and was distinctly narrower. And then a remarkable thing began to happen. Day after day, my nurse would pull back my dressing, and I would watch as this great wound, in the slow, patient way of all natural things, gradually became a long thin hairline scar. And I, a physician, was not in control of this. It was humbling. Yet, I certainly had a front row seat. So do you.

So perhaps what is useful to remember is that the tenacity towards life is our birthright. It exists in every one of our cells. The Will to Live is present even in the most elderly and the tiniest of human beings. The power of the life force in those two little green blades of grass is there in us all.

Based on a story in *Kitchen Table Wisdom (Riverhead)*, 1996.
Dr. Remen has retold the story for *I Am with You*.

NONSENSE

Sue Glader

I have an innate desire to make sense of things. I'm not a scientist or anything, but I do like order in my little corner of the world.

Cancer is not orderly. It is, by definition, uncontrolled growth. And it was dropped into my lap at age thirty-three, when I was in the midst of my own un-orderly new mother situation. Hans had recently celebrated his first birthday, and was tottering on unsteady legs and uttering interesting noises in an attempt to communicate. I had no idea what I was doing, like most new mothers, but I was doing it nevertheless.

It wasn't a good time for cancer.

I couldn't make any sense of why I got it in the first place — what I did or didn't do. I suppose my desire to accept some sort of blame is counter to getting on with the job of healing, but I couldn't help it.

I was diagnosed with breast cancer during the month of October, totally on trend. There were endless advertisements and feature stories in magazines and on television, and ladies walking through my town in full pink regalia for fundraising walks. Breast cancer surrounded me, literally.

My mother, who comes from New England pilgrim stock,

commingles "chin up, let's get going" resolve with perhaps just the right amount of avoidance. I followed her lead. Appointments were made and met, surgery and chemo and radiation ensued. I joined a support group. I took my meds. My hair re-emerged.

I just did what needed to be done.

But I was hardly done with cancer. I wanted to—I needed to—untangle the "what-the-hell-just-happened-to-me?" tsunami of feelings that washed over me post-treatment. As a woman of action, I decided that creating something around cancer felt right. I wanted to turn the tables and make something lasting, beautiful, and, above all else, helpful, in those early moments when everything just seems to be coming too fast to digest.

As a writer by trade, and a young mother at the time, I focused my attention close to home. I wrote from what I had experienced: kids looking at my baldness with big eyes and silence. What emerged, I entitled *Nowhere Hair*, a picture book to help explain a loved one's cancer diagnosis to kids ages three to ten.

The book is honest yet decidedly upbeat. I wanted to convey a sense of dignity and style. After all, we are the same confident, beautiful, loving, stylish women we were before cancer. We just don't happen to have hair at that moment. I also did not want to portray the woman as scary-looking or an emotional mess.

Edith Buenen, a fashion illustrator from the Netherlands, is the primary reason the book has such a positive feel. Even in the pages that talk about the hardest things ("It makes me scared that she is sick. I want her well right now. She says, 'Be patient, little one.' That seems so hard somehow."), her pictures are lyrical and calming. Yes indeed, mommy is cranky sometimes and wiped out and on the couch. But she is still a mommy first and foremost, filled with love for children. The book explains that children can't catch cancer, and didn't cause it to happen. It ends with the universal message that what is inside of us matters far more than how we look on the outside. That's how I made sense of the nonsense of having cancer.

This little book has spanned the globe, helping big people open up a pathway for communication with the little people in their lives. It is a small part of me—how I see the world, how I face adversity, how I choose to be remembered—that will always be around. And I like that idea.

WHAT WORKED FOR ME

Firstly, mothering my little one-year-old Hans with all my heart. Focusing on him helped me to remember what I was fighting for. Then, embracing the baldness, both physical and metaphorical. I often went full Telly Savalas around town, but also entered therapy for the first time in my life (thought it would be a couple of days, and ended up going for a couple of years . . .). Then, believing in my mother's mantra that "This too shall pass." And finally, planning a victory lap when all the treatment was over: first Yosemite, then Italy.

WHO NEEDS BREASTS, ANYWAY?

Molly Ivins

Having breast cancer is massive amounts of no fun. First they mutilate you; then they poison you; then they burn you. I have been on blind dates better than that.

One of the first things you notice is that people treat you differently when they know you have it. The hushed tone in which they inquire, "How are you?" is unnerving. If I had answered honestly during 90 percent of the nine months I spent in treatment, I would have said, "If it weren't for being constipated, I'd be fine." In fact, even chemotherapy is not nearly as hard as it once was, although it still made all my hair fall out. My late friend Jocelyn Gray found the ultimate proof that there is no justice: "Not just my hair, but my eyebrows, my eyelashes—every hair on my body has fallen out, except for these goddam little mustaches at the corner of my mouth I have always hated."

Another thing you get as a cancer patient is a lot of football-coach patter. "You can beat this; you can win; you're strong; you're tough; get psyched." I suspect that cancer doesn't give a rat's ass whether you have a positive mental attitude. It just sits in there multiplying away, whether you are admirably stoic or weeping and wailing. The only reason to have a positive mental attitude is that it makes life better. It doesn't cure cancer.

My friend Judy Curtis demanded totally uncritical support from everyone around her. "I smoked and drank through the whole thing," she says. "And I hated the lady from the American Cancer Society." My role model.

The late Alice Trillin wrote some brilliant essays on being a cancer patient, and I found her theory of "the good student" especially helpful. When you are not doing well at cancer—barfing and getting bad blood tests and generally not sailing through the whole thing with grace and panache—you have a tendency to think, Help, I'm flunking cancer, as though it were your fault. Your doctor also tends to look at you as though he is disappointed. Especially if you start to die on him.

You don't get through this without friends. Use them. Call them, especially other women who have been through it. People like to help. They like to be able to do something for you. Let them. You will also get sick of talking about cancer. One way to hold down the solicitous calls is to give your friends a regular update by email, if you have it. If you work, I recommend that you keep right on doing so (unless you hate your job). Most companies are quite good about giving you time off when you need it, and working keeps you from sitting around and worrying.

Losing a part of a breast or all of one or both has, obviously, serious psychological consequences. Your self-image, your sense of yourself as a woman, your sense of your sexual attractiveness are going to be rocked, whether or not you have enough sense to realize that tits aren't that important. I am one of those people who are out of touch with their emotions. I tend to treat my emotions like unpleasant relatives—a long-distance call once or twice or year is more than enough. If I got in touch with them, they might come to stay. My friend Mercedes Peña made me get in touch with my emotions just before I had a breast cut off. Just as I suspected, they were awful. "How do you Latinas do this—all the time in touch with your emotions?" I asked her. "That's why we take siestas," she replied.

As a final indignity, I have just flunked breast reconstruction. Bad enough that I went through all that pain for the sake of vanity, but then I got a massive infection and had to have both implants taken out. I'm embarrassed about it, although my chief cancer mentor, Marlyn Schwartz (who went to the Palm for lunch after every chemo session), has forbidden this particular emotion. So now I'm just a happy, flat-chested woman.

Originally appeared in *Time*, 2002

I WATCHED MY MOM REINVENT HERSELF

Sophia Kercher

She surprised me after she lost all of her hair.

My mom had the kind of hair that seemed to grow larger by the hour. It was so magnificent and massive that I thought it must have held secrets. I could always spot her from yards away—a big brunette mass attached to a feminine form. When she was growing up, she told me, she would lay her head on a flat surface while a family member ironed her dark brown curls until they were smooth. It took an hour because her hair was so thick. Mornings in the house I grew up in meant the hum of a blow dryer and the mysterious smells of smoothing serums and hairsprays.

My mom was diagnosed with breast cancer and told she would have to undergo chemotherapy treatment when I was twenty-six. I cried hardest at the thought of my mother without her hair. When I was a teenager, she lent me her curling iron as if she were passing on a baton to womanhood. She is a raven-haired Snow White beauty, while I'm more of a California blonde, but we have the same overly abundant tresses, and we both feel they are our most attractive traits. I couldn't imagine her without them.

After my mom completed the first month of chemo, her

hair surprised us by remaining stubbornly on her head. I prayed that she would be the exception to the treatment's horrible side effects. But, after another round of chemo, that proved not to be the case.

My family was traveling across the country to go to my grandmother's funeral when my mom's hair started falling out by the handfuls. What was once her defining feature became little dark nests resting in the hotel's sink. My sister and I mourned both for the loss of our sweet ninety-three-year-old grandmom and for our mother's locks.

My mom startled us with her bravery, though. When we returned home to northern California, she immediately had her hairdresser shave off the remaining wisps on her head. She emerged from the hair salon completely bareheaded, looking fragile—like a newly hatched bird. For the first time, I noticed how pretty her hazel eyes were.

She no longer spent hours primping in the bathroom. She no longer chided me for not brushing my hair, or leaving the house without makeup. But she had not given up. We added to her collection of hats and went shopping for dangly earrings and daring lipsticks, which she said helped her feel more feminine. I began to see her in a new light. I admired my mom's courage as she announced her illness to our Sacramento neighbors.

I went with her to pick out a wig, and although she was battling nausea, she was excited. "I can totally reinvent myself," she told me. "I can be anyone I want."

She fell in love with a rock 'n' roll style mullet, and I was partial to a red bob. I made her try on my own hairdo—long, sun-bleached locks. She felt like a babe, she said. I told her she looked like a preteen. She laughed. We settled on a reasonably priced shoulder-length brunette style with red highlights, and it suited her so much that people thought she had just gotten a new haircut.

But the new wig was itchy and tight on her head. She joked about tattooing the words "cancer sucks" on her bald head. She didn't wear her new faux-hairdo much, and I was glad she didn't. Around the house, her head was bare as she stirred a pot of hot water with fresh ginger to calm chemo's side effects, or watched as my dad did. When we took short walks, she wore a newsboy cap, which made her appear much younger than her fifty-six years.

Her hair had been such a dramatic feature that few people in the neighborhood recognized her without it. She didn't tell many of them who she was. Her illness quieted her in a way I wasn't used to. It no longer took ten minutes to leave the grocery store, because she no longer told the checkout clerk things like, "I love pasta, I can eat it everyday. Maybe it's because I grew up in Italy? Have you been to Rome? No? My daughter lived there for half a year, and she had at least three Italian boyfriends. But it was hard for her—so many people! Still, you have to go to Europe. Why haven't you been to Europe?"

Then her hair finally grew back, and for the first time, I saw its natural gray hue. The salt-and-pepper Annie Lennox-short style suited her. "You're really lucky," her artist friend Sal told her. "You have such a great-shaped head."

The silver in her hair lit up her eyes. She looked hip. My sister and I begged her to keep the hairstyle. People stopped her in the streets to tell her how much they liked her look. She had a difficult time accepting the compliments. She wanted to tell them the closely cropped hair wasn't by choice. It wasn't until it grew back longer—silky and fine—and she colored it back to brown that she felt more at ease walking around the neighborhood with our dogs. She started talking to strangers again—sometimes in Italian.

For Halloween, she loaded it with gel and shaped it into a Mohawk. I barely recognized her. But, by then, it didn't matter, I was used to that.

Originally appeared in *Reimagine* magazine, 2014

WHAT I DID DURING THOSE FREAK-OUT NIGHTS

When both my parents—my anchors in the world—had to deal with cancer, there were many nights spent fraught with worry. My antidote to those panicky nights was books. I drowned myself in other worlds, revisiting Truman Capote's Breakfast at Tiffany's *in which I could transport myself to 1940s Manhattan. There, I became transfixed with Holly Golightly who was every bit as lost as I, but she knew how to communicate it. I love her line: "I'll never get used to anything. Anybody that does, they might as well be dead."*

I let myself cry while reading Lorrie Moore's stories in Birds of America, *many of them about what it is to be a woman who feels truly alone. I read Junot Diaz's brilliant novel* The Brief Wondrous Life of Oscar Wao *and my troubles dwarfed as I learned about the Dominican Republic's violent past through the main character, Oscar, and his family history. And those were just a few of my reading selections.*

My dad had read stories to me every night from age two to ten. And when my mother was sick, I read aloud to her, so we could both transport ourselves somewhere else — if only for a few moments.

EAT WHATEVER YOU CAN
Terri White Tate

Eating has always been one of my favorite pastimes. Then oral cancer robbed me of a large portion of my tongue and lower jaw. Surgery for twenty-four hours failed to craft a new mouth from my transplanted hipbone. A titanium bar was installed to replace my jaw, and then it came loose during radiation.

Learning to eat with my modified mouth has been one of the major challenges of my life since cancer. But I am nothing if not a committed eater!

While I will never again bite into a big red apple or eat corn on the cob, I manage to nourish myself very well and, once again, take tremendous pleasure from food. What got me through? During the really rough times, the doctors told me to eat whatever I could. I had always wanted doctors to say that to me! I should have been more specific about the circumstances.

Friends brought over food, even when I couldn't eat it. Friends brought over food when I could eat it, like custard. Friends sat with me, however long it took me to eat. Meals go faster now, but I am still the last one at any table. My dear friends now sit across the dinner table from me without fear of getting sprayed with food bits.

Blending is my secret weapon. You can blend almost anything. After lots of blended meals, I now appreciate the texture of food almost as much as the taste.

And, as one of my friends says, with a smile we share, "Isn't it ironic that you can eat all desserts?"

THE THINGS THAT HELPED ME THROUGH

My kids and wanting to see them grow up
My fervent desire to be a grandmother
Time in Sausalito
More and better friends than I could have fathomed
The discovery of my Guides—gentle inner advisors
A loyal—at the time—husband
Ice cream—especially soft serve
Shamanic journeys
My sister
Roxicett (liquid morphine)
A Master Mind Group
A Course in Miracles
The Daily Word
Late Night with David Letterman
Bette Midler music
God's will

LIVINGLY DYING

Marcy Westerling

Dying inevitably follows living. What makes for a good death in a just and sustainable world? I think about this a lot these days. Four years ago, at age fifty, I was diagnosed with late-stage ovarian cancer. Active and fit, it took a collapsed lung and two broken ribs before I realized I had a big problem, the ultimate challenge of life: facing my own death.

In the first weeks after learning I was terminally ill, I wondered, *Will I face this in my heart or in my head? In my head, it is a storyline I can make interesting, wise, and abstract. In my heart, it is a constant tremor radiating from my stomach.* As the first months of terror subsided, I began to adapt to my "new normal." My medical team advised, "You must start living as if the next three months are your last. When you are still alive at the close, make a new three-month plan." I resolved to hope and dream and build in smaller allocations of time.

I made huge shifts in my life, severing two critical anchor points. I moved to the city from the small town that had been my home for twenty-five years—my isolated existence in the woods seemed too daunting for the emotional swings of terminal cancer. I retired from the organization I had founded and that had been my life's work for eighteen years. I knew the long hours and stress of the job I loved would deplete the strength I needed for cancer treatment.

I qualified for Social Security disability income, thanks to the government's "compassion clause," and this got me Medicare two and a half years later. I stepped into my new life determined to live as long as possible. I decided I would live to be seventy-two years old, nineteen years longer than the statistics predicted, and an age I found acceptable to die.

It is estimated that one in three people in the United States will receive a cancer diagnosis at some point in life. Some people die quickly. Others diagnosed as terminal continue to live fully even while facing a death sentence. A friend who had watched her mother die of cancer remarked on my vivacity. In the fifteen years since her mother's death, there have been advancements that make the devastating side effects of treatment more tolerable. Still, it has taken me years after my diagnosis to re-embrace the commitments that populate a full life.

I chafe at being invisible as a person with cancer. I am a lifelong feminist and community organizer. I believe in breaking silence and sharing truth. I pass as "normal"—healthy, white, slender, and heterosexual (having a husband helps). I have lived a life of privilege. For now, I don't look or feel like I'm dying. I am just terminally ill.

Recently, I was reminded of the great Rachel Carson. She hid the pain of her end-stage cancer to keep her *Silent Spring* message of environmental degradation alive in Congress and mainstream conversation back in 1964.

In 2014, I can choose to be visible. I have a tattoo on my

wrist declaring me a "Cancer Warrior." I sport buttons saying "Cancer Sucks." I pedal everywhere, slowly, on a bike that announces "Cancer on Board." I defy every attempt to limit me to my diagnosis as I dare the world to ignore it.

But sometimes I feel I am as isolated in shouting about my diagnosis as Rachel Carson was in secrecy. I look so good that observers may well conclude that the sign on my bike, the buttons on my bags, even the tattoo on my wrist represent strength and survival. Public or private, silent or loud, the outcomes are the same. Disease creates isolation and barriers from the world of the well. A friend with terminal cancer notes, "We cause discomfort to some because we are living, living in acute awareness of our impending death, living in pain but living as fully as we can while we are dying. Should we lock ourselves away in a figurative darkened room so as not to chance disturbing the hale and hearty with thoughts of death?"

People say odd things when they attempt to comfort the terminally ill while avoiding their own fears. "We are all terminally ill. You just know it." I more than "know it" as my weary veins dodge yet another dose of chemotherapy, toxic poison that will bring me to my knees with exhaustion, nausea, and brain fog while hopefully keeping me alive a while longer.

While the statistics gave me little hope, real people with cancer provide inspiration. They look normal and live well. They laugh, watch TV, and travel. They haven't stopped living, even as medical appointments, surgeries, treatments, and side effects disrupt their days.

I sought out other women living with a pink slip from life and discovered how hard it is for us to find each other. Medical privacy laws don't help. Advocacy groups are often Internet- or hospital-based, but not everyone flourishes in those settings. Eventually, I created my own support circle of other women with terminal cancer. The group is called "It's a Dying Shame," and the outreach flyer states, "Our goal is to explore the rich and peculiar territory of facing our own deaths. Together we can mine the humor, strangeness, and beauty of a life turned upside down. Join us for tea down the rabbit hole." Our group meetings provide a cherished time to speak our truth without taking on the emotions of friends and family.

People often say to the terminally ill, "You are so stoic, so graceful. I could never handle this so well." Perhaps not. The truth is you have no idea how well or badly we, the dying, handle it. Kim, diagnosed as terminal three years ago at age thirty-four, says, "Each day can vary greatly. Is it a doctor appointment day? Scan day? A day of total rest and relaxation? A day that the thought of me dying before age forty leaves me immobilized, weeping in bed, and tightly grasping a heating pad? In a month's time, I go through all of these typical days. And then some."

Social media also allows us to communicate with new ease about approaching death. Thousands follow Lisa Adams' blog, where she describes every aspect of the medical and emotional realities of facing death as she copes with raising a young family. She doesn't make it look easy or pretty. Lisa and other dying bloggers offer a view of pain that is normally rarely witnessed and ask that people with terminal cancer be seen as more than "courageous." *Guardian* columnist Emma Keller and her husband chided Adams for over-sharing. I think that those who condemn our process are distancing themselves from Lisa—and

80

me—and from the reality of protracted death.

The current rules of polite conversation make the journey toward death more challenging. One woman said to me, "It is like we are standing in a different room." We are avoided or jollied up. ("You look so good you can't be terminally ill" is the most hated and common of compliments.) These approaches insulate people in our culture from sitting with death, sadly but comfortably.

When people with terminal diagnoses communicate about their experience, it may make their walking toward death more doable. I cannot think of subjects better suited for full honesty than birth and death.

There is a trend to reframe some terminal cancers as a chronic disease, perhaps to avoid mention of death, to give hope, or because some terminal diseases are becoming more manageable over the years. One woman in her forties rejected that label after six years in treatment: "For most people, it makes sense to make plans beyond one month at a time, but even that short a time-frame can turn out to be optimistic for me. Unexpected side effects catch up with me; treatments that we thought were working cease to work months earlier than expected, and suddenly we are thrust again into making life-and-death decisions, lacking any real information about what may—or may not—buy me even a few more months of life. Making plans in this context becomes almost a joke. Something about this state that I live in seems really different to me from what I think of as chronic illness. It is more like a slow dying process, during which I get to live."

I have noticed many of us with terminal cancer are of good

cheer and even invigorated by having no presumption of longevity. We have little choice but to live in the moment; something many talk about, but few can manage. When you live treatment to treatment and test result to test result, there is less room for distraction by petty stresses. We can't expect to live another year, but if we do survive one year, or five, or ten, we consider ourselves very lucky. My mandate is to live with the shadow of death seated comfortably on one shoulder—I rarely forget, but I often dismiss, my new companion.

I have made a certain peace with leaving this world, a peace experienced only after pondering what I might do, where I might be, what I might become after I die. I live in a culture that offers few views of what happens after death—it is either the end (humus for the ages), or it is some mythic version of heaven and hell. Neither option works for me. I imagine my next world as Peter Pan did, "To die will be an awfully big adventure," even if his image of death is more boisterous than mine.

Weeks after my diagnosis, before relocating to the city, I sat in the spring sunshine by a creek at our homestead while my sweetie did the chores I couldn't do post-surgery. This was a favorite spot of mine. The chickens made comforting clucks in their enclosure to my right while the ducks quacked comically in the pasture to my left. The warmth of the sun reached every nook of my body. I was surrounded by so much that I loved—the tears I cried were happy ones. Couldn't this be my heaven?

Today, I live in a lovely neighborhood, in a lovely house surrounded by pleasures that don't take away the sorrow of departure. My life stays filled with joy and meaning as well as sadness and grief. I am livingly dying. Dying is woven into the reality of living. Neither is easy. But just as we live as a community, let's face death as a community too.

Originally appeared in *Yes! Magazine*, 2014

WHAT GOT ME THROUGH, FRONTLINE?

I dramatically altered my life, moving in with friends who took care of everything, and allowed my husband and me the space to process this unexpected reality. Humor—laughing even when crying. People crawling into bed with me.

What keeps me going, as I enter my fifth year of treatment: accepting treatment and the many chores of surviving treatment as my job. Helping others cope keeps my woes in perspective.

GOING DALLAS BUYERS CLUB

Anonymous

I was diagnosed a year ago. I have a seventeen-year-old son who I adore, so failure to heal has never been an option for me.

My treatment and surgery went very well, so we were shocked in March when we found that I had not gone into remission. My doctor told me that the disease was now chronic, that I would be on chemo for the rest of my life, and did not offer me much hope.

What I heard was that I needed a different protocol—one that could get me into remission. My beloved family and friends stayed strong and helped me keep the faith. My therapist made house calls.

My doctor opposed any treatment that was not in his study trials. I can understand that, but to my way of thinking, this was the time to experiment, because his protocol didn't have a good prognosis. So I went *Dallas Buyers Club* on him. I called all over the country looking for information and answers; that's how I met Nancy.

Nancy told me not to give up on Doxil—she had had good results with it. She also said, "You need a doctor who is taking care of you." That hit home.

Just by chance, my doctor was replaced by a doctor who brought joy and hope to his work, and he was open to all medicines. That's when things got interesting! I started taking Frankincense, which has a reputation for working well with chemo, killing only the cancer cells, and has no side effects. I also added two Chinese mushrooms, astragalus and coriolus, recommended by an alternative medicine doctor at my hospital, and by the Arizona Institute of Health.

I doubled my efforts on the nutrition front—I was already an organic vegetarian, with no caffeine, alcohol, or sugar in my diet, but I went primarily raw vegan with no sugar at all, not even fruit.

I enjoyed massages three hours a week, with essential oils, given by a dedicated friend.

I spent every second I could outdoors in nature.

After three months on this protocol, I knew I was getting better. My son and doctor and I are overjoyed by how great my recent CT scan looks. We're talking about the possibility of my being in remission in three months, and going forward after remission. I'm so grateful and proud to be here, at peak health.

You can do this. Be as flexible and determined and resilient as a fire hose. Find a doctor who will take care of you.

With love, hugs, and encouragement to each and all of you, my sisters and brothers!

WHAT KEPT THE FRENZY AT BAY

1. *Help. I asked for help. I asked everybody, all the time. I'm a giver by nature. Receiving was a challenge! But I did it.*

2. *Community. My community came together to save my life and heal me. I don't have a partner and feared I would not be able to manage emotionally or physically, but I was not by myself at all for the first thirty days of my treatment, when I was too ill to move. After that, I had people there whenever I needed them, for over a year. Friends and family flew in from all over the country, all the time. All of them had lost a family member or best friend to cancer, so they were unbelievably empathetic and fiercely loving. I believe the intensity of their commitment inspired them all. My best friend organized the whole process; it was a second job for her for a year.*

3. *My sister meditated with me during treatments. That was the best support.*

4. *Several people got up and stood between death and me.*

5. *My son was there for me. We built our courage together. FIGHT LIKE A MOTHER.*

6. *I was inspired by the warriors I know who live life to the fullest, despite the loss of limbs and issues like PTSD. Before I knew them, I thought that if I were to lose my legs, I would be entitled to end my life if I wanted. After spending time with them, I knew if I suffered an injury like that, I would have to start doing triathlons. Under their influence, and because of my son, when I got diagnosed, I said, AW, HELL NO!*

Also under their inspiration, I worked to spread love, joy, hope, happiness, and inspiration in my hospital. The doctors, nurses, technicians, and receptionists are so kind and supportive. Most of us patients look and act so depressed and despairing. I did everything I could think of to return their kindness and build my hospital into a place of healing, not despair.

7. The Dalai Lama healing chants. I played them throughout my treatments. The Dalai Lama knows how to bring the world into harmony—one person at a time.

8. I meditated with the mantras of Thich Nhat Hahn three times a day, while lying in bed.

9. Nicki Minaj song: "Massive Attack." I played that throughout my treatments, too.

10. Trace Adkins song: "Tough People Do" says, "Tough people keep on fighting like they don't know how to lose."

11. For a long time, I did no things at a time. After that I did one thing at a time. One thing at a time is AWESOME.

12. SPREADING LOVE when I was too chemo-ed out to work. I spent my waking hours calling people to tell them how much I loved them. After a while, I realized I had a new job.

13. I got off the axis of evil—genetically modified and processed foods, sugar, and white flour.

14. I cleared my life of traumas I couldn't fix. No TV news, newspapers, depressing books, friends who depress me.

15. I reframed all my fears into adamant affirmations of life.

16. I prayed, and I asked everyone to pray for me. I called and emailed and reminded them I needed it.

17. *I got close to my sister. Very happy about that.*

18. *TINTIN: I read Tintin cartoons in French by the hour in bed. In French, I was not sick.*

19. *ORGASMS: It's a life-affirming action.*

20. *BABY MEDICINE: One of my best girlfriends brought over her new baby every week for hours. This was the best medicine!*

21. *HEALING THURSDAYS: She and I and one other girlfriend invented Healing Thursdays—a stress-free day when I only do healing things.*

22. *I learned to become my best advocate. My cousins taught me how to research and ask my doctors questions and have a friend write them down, in case I forgot everything the doctors said out of fear.*

23. *When I switched chemos to a tougher medicine, I decided it was necessary to reinvent myself as a superhero. With the help of the girlfriend above, I dressed up and she photographed me as a 1970s Blaxploitation superstar.*

24. *One of my cousins gave me* Kitchen Table Wisdom *by Rachel Naomi Remen, M.D., a must read. One thing I learned in it was how doctors and nurses don't have therapeutic support for dealing with injury and death. During the bad times, I stayed calm and strong in their offices and saved the hysterical weeping for my community. It really helped our doctor-patient relationship.*

25. *HOMEOPATHIC MEDICINE: From Rescue Remedy for sleep to Traumeel for pain, which got me off the pain meds, to*

some specialty prescriptions like "speaking my truth and getting it out of the body."

26. *I let go.*

FINDING FLATWATER
Mark Garza

So many people are affected by one cancer diagnosis. And each of them needs help and support to deal with this terrible news. I know this, because, a few years ago, my leader, my inspiration, and my coach (we called him Dad) told us, "I have stage IV cancer."

Dad had made an odd request. He had gathered all four of his children at a table in the living room to talk. We hadn't done this, outside of the holidays, since we were in grade school. Now in our thirties, we lived all over the country, so we knew the news was going to be big. Nothing can prepare a person for the gravity of the message we heard that day. People all over the world are hearing this news now, every day. "I have cancer."

Everyone reacted differently. My oldest brother moved quickly to tears. My sisters sat in silence, and then moved over to help my brother. My mother seemed to bear most of the weight of this news. And me? Well, it was as if all motion, for a moment, ceased. I could not help but look around and take mental pictures of the scene. I will never forget that day. The sounds of my brother's crying soon flooded back in. The hands of time started to turn again. We shared paper-thin words intended to ameliorate our concerns and put everyone at ease.

But it was far from easy. I share my story with hopes that the work my father has inspired and the lesson he taught me will spread through thousands of hearts and minds. My goal is to empower people across the world to think more about their minds, the importance of mental health, and what counseling, exercise, and mindfulness can do to help overcome the challenges of a cancer diagnosis.

Family turbulence followed the news of my father's cancer. Like a boulder crashing into a beautiful calm mountain lake, waves were all around us, and our boats seemed to be drifting apart. My mother and my father soon separated. After four decades together, they severed their ties. I read that nearly 12 percent of marriages end in divorce or separation after a spouse develops cancer. And so I knew that we were not alone and not unique in any way when it came to feeling like the walls were closing in.

The mental disruption struck us all, not just my mom and dad. For my family, and even our close friends, it wasn't just the cancer. It was the news of the cancer. Our minds were under attack, and everything seemed shaky. Without a clear and balanced mind, nothing was clear. Even the path to answers seemed foggy.

Late in 2009, something really unexpected happened. Stand up paddle boarding leapt from the coasts to the inner waterways of America. A friend gave me his board as a payment for some consulting services, and it turned out to be the wind that cleared the fog for me. Every day, I would set my alarm for 5:45 A.M., load up my board, and head downtown to get on a small stretch of the Colorado River known as Lady Bird Lake, in Austin. I was one of the only people on the water, with a paddle in hand, gliding across the surface with a chilly breeze in my face and a newfound sense of calm and peacefulness drenching my heart and mind. It became my "church on the water," and I started to see life in a new way. Always one to recognize the importance of exercise, I hadn't expected what I now refer to as "accidentally meditating"—the perfect calm, birds chirping, cool air, and even an actual light fog layer on the water being cut by the nose of the board, creating beautiful spinning wisps of air on either side of me.

My mind and soul began to elevate. I soon found myself on the water most mornings and, when I wasn't, I met with my trainer in the gym. I shed twenty-five pounds, the right way, and I felt more and more empowered to take on any challenge. My mind had become more centered, and I felt great about being there for my father, for my family. Naturally, I began to feel like I had a story to share with them. It started small, but my goal was to lead by example and show them how to take control of their minds, and to change their perception of what was happening in our lives. In the end, that's just it: how you perceive your situation has everything to do with how you handle it. But even with all of the growth I was feeling, something was missing, and I knew it.

I sensed that I needed some professional guidance, but, never having visited a therapist before, I didn't know where to begin. Getting care was still a mystery. I had lived with mostly good news, triumphs, happy successes, and a positive outlook in my life. I was afraid that getting help would mean I was weak. The stigma around seeing a therapist had me thinking, *If I go, does that mean I have a "shrink"?* It didn't matter, and I decided to take the leap.

My initial session was everything I wanted and needed: a person who could listen to me, a person who knew all the right things to ask, and somehow made me feel as though everything I was saying was not new, not confusing. To be honest, I remember feeling at one point like she had known me for years, and somehow totally understood where I was coming from. This was just a first meeting, and I was already changed. But what came next was going to change the lives of hundreds of people over the next couple of years, and I could never have expected that.

After just one hour-long session, I walked out feeling like a new champion and a cheerleader for psychotherapy. It was as if I wanted to grab a megaphone, ready to shout the news that there was a powerful tool out there in the war against cancer and everyone needed to know about it. But I was still not sure that those who needed it could afford it, especially those who were hit by a wallet-draining cancer diagnosis. That was it—the "aha" moment, if you will—when I decided that I would spread the news. I had found my purpose, to share the message that getting help for your mind was not for crazy people. It was for healthy people.

And that, in the end, is why I share my story—to work towards breaking down this stigma against mental health support and therapy, and to help provide access to help for those in need. My transformation led me to see how deeply the mind and body and all of our actions are tied together. I not only felt the weight of the cancer diagnosis across my family, but I also found ways to work through the fear, the confusion, and the stress—by looking to others while digging deep inside.

Every year, in the hot June Texas sun, droves of people come together to paddle twenty-one miles on stand up paddle boards, with mental might, to raise hundreds of thousands of dollars to foot the bill for so many others in need. This event is hosted by The Flatwater Foundation, which I founded to provide mental health support for families in need affected by a cancer diagnosis. Flatwater looks to change the way people think about getting help. That's what it's all about—calming the waters while helping others.

My father overcame his cancer for years, but finally ran out of time and passed in November of 2013. Because of his diagnosis, and the mental challenges faced by my family, I saw the huge hole in the circle of care for those facing cancer. I call my organization "flatwater" because one diagnosis causes so many waves in every direction. We work to bring those families back to the serenity of calm, flat water, so everyone can focus on overcoming cancer, not mental imbalance.

Here's to hoping you can find your own flatwater.

WHAT HELPED ME

Getting outdoors in nature to clear my mind has always been the key to getting through hard times. Cancer is no different. When faced with my father's terminal diagnosis, I found myself on a paddle board at 6 A.M., awakening the senses. I found myself taking on new tasks and keeping myself busy, which, to many, can be a negative way to deal with stress. The projects I created became a nonprofit dedicated to helping other people who are dealing with cancer get access to mental health support. In a sense, I was able to get through it by helping others get through it.

CONNECTIONS

"The universe took my tightly closed hand, pried it open, and placed your hand inside saying, 'See, there is hope.'"
—Shauna Shapiro

LIFE IS A JOURNEY, NOT A DESTINATION

Anonymous

My therapist does not get it. She says things like, "Well, you just have to endure," or, "You are asking me to fix something I can't fix." I don't expect her to fix anything, but when I start to lose my mojo, when my fighting spirit lags, where else do I turn? When I stare, every single day, at life's final destination, how on earth do I appreciate life as a journey?

Being on the cancer track, I get to ask these questions.

We cancer folk—call us survivors, call us warriors, call us in remission—we know that there will be a destination for us. For some of us, the little cells will mutate some more; the little cells will someday overpower the other cells. The journey for us, once we have heard that news, is figuring out how to live with the known destination.

Most women won't want to hear my story, because I am the one who was supposed to be cured. I had less than one centimeter of invasive cancer twenty years ago. I had "the best pathology ever seen." But I'm no longer in the safe zone; my cancer that was cured has defied all of the odds and come back.

Now, to put this in context, I remember being told by doctors that I would die within a year if I had a child. That child is now a healthy, happy seventeen-year-old, and I'm still living well.

I remember being told to forget I ever had cancer because it wouldn't come back. Just to put it all behind me. Hah, that was a good one! I have had my body chopped and carved up so much that I have no body shame left. Sound familiar? Well, you are welcome to join me in the hot tub any old time!

I have had to forge my own journey. Some days, that is simply putting one foot in front of the other for as long as possible. Only it doesn't feel simple, to keep walking strong while acknowledging that there is a destination, a journey's end. That is the razor's edge of a cancer diagnosis—you can lean toward happiness and hope, or fear and futility. Sometimes I lean in all directions at once, but the goal is always to lean towards hope!

My journey is mine; your journey is yours. But the "big C" has given us a path so tied to impermanence that we get to be brave, like it or not. Walk through it with me, journey with me. I need you. Because my therapist just doesn't get it.

WHAT HELPED ME THROUGH THE DARK HOURS

The dark hours . . . nighttime can be really tough for us cancer folk. After twenty years of fighting the "big C," I'm still not sure if I can offer much beyond letting you know you are not alone, if sleep is elusive.

I think nights can be so hard because our busy-ness stops. My cancer buddies and I talk about 2:00 A.M.s . . . for us, this is the time we wake up and can't keep those scary thoughts at bay. Despite our best intentions and convictions, some nights, all our fears come rushing in. For parents, it may be worries about our children and how they will be without us. For all of us, we may worry about the treatment decisions: Did I choose the right treatment? How will I face the eventual challenges that the disease may bring?

Those nights—after treatment ends, or before doctors' visits, tests or scans—can be really tough. We may toss and turn, trying to play out scenarios in our heads. So much depends on these results. Our realities hang in the balance.

For each of us, these challenging nights will differ, but when they strike, please remember that you will get through. The dark hours are hard, for you are human after all. So when they strike, please try to remember they will pass and most fears seem more manageable with the light of day.

WHY MY BFFS ARE MY CHORE WHORES
Aisling Carroll

I sit on my living room floor, lean my head back against my green couch, and try to focus. Squint-eyed, I gaze up in awe at Katy, who sits above me and holds my cell phone like a bolt of lightning while she effortlessly dials Comcast. I think she might be a superhero.

I have been Internet- and TV-less since Comcast cut me off two days ago. They had left me half a dozen messages. "Hello, this is Comcast calling. Please return our call at 1-800-COMCAST," said the customer service representative in a sweet and high-pitched tone. But then her voice dropped perilously. "This is not a sales call."

In the middle of a horrid few days of near blackouts, calling Comcast was not a possibility. But as soon as Katy walked in, she offered to sort it.

As she victoriously puts my phone down, I feel a potent mix of relief and gratefulness well up in my chest. And I can't help but wonder, "Why is she still friends with me?"

When I was diagnosed with ovarian cancer at thirty-two, more than six years ago, this was not how I pictured our friendship "growing" after cancer. Before I started chemo, I imagined Katy and me taking leisurely early spring walks along a beach. As if recovering from a cold, I would be bundled up in a large checkered scarf and a woolen hat. Katy would wear a cotton cardigan.

Meandering through the sand, we would swap talk of our usual, day-to-day dramas for the weightier topics. "Life lessons" and "philosophies of living" and other *Tuesdays with Morrie* insights would dominate our discourse. I would be wise. Katy would be eager.

There have been no walks along the beach. No enlightened teachings. No radically different life philosophies touted. Instead, Katy has received lists of tasks to complete, tasks that are sometimes physically beyond me. Call Dr. Milano's office. Pick up prescriptions. Look for juicer.

As well as my friends' willingness to be my chore whores, what I prize most about my friends is their ability to:

Fetch and forget. When you're stuck in your bed unable to do things for yourself, such as grab some Ensure from the fridge or remove a blanket, you have to alert your family and friends for help. My way of getting my friend Jeremy's attention, when he was out in the living room, was to throw a tennis ball against my bedroom wall. Jeremy would hear the thump and scamper in. One evening, when my friend Ruth was at my bedside, and I was wired on steroids, I decided to show her how the system worked. I threw the tennis ball and Jeremy promptly came into the bedroom. "You called?" he said. "Oh, yeah, but I don't need anything," I responded matter-of-factly. "I was just showing Ruth our system." The fact that he didn't hurl the tennis ball at my head is remarkable. And that he still considers me a friend is testament to his power to forget.

Escape with me. In the early days of treatment, escapism meant spending hours with my friends watching *Arrested Development* and reading aloud from Matt Groening's *The Big Book of Hell*. We cracked ourselves up. A few months later, however, things got more serious, and we shifted to escapism in the literal sense. A case in point was when my friend Carlina and I arrived at the hospital for my routine check between chemo sessions. Placing her fingers on my forehead, the nurse said, "You seem a little warm. I think you should come into this room here while I go get a thermometer." Crestfallen, I knew this meant she would keep me in this hospital room for days. I decided to be the empowered cancer patient I kept reading about. I snuck out of the room, grabbed Carlina (who was sitting outside in the hallway), and buoyantly walked out the big front doors. The best part was Carlina not saying, mid-breakout, "Do you really think this is such a good idea?"

Protractedly nod. Listening is indeed an act of love. For me, being able to spill with friends who nod and commiserate makes me feel less separate in my sickness. For my friends, I am sure hearing me say, "It's been a brutal few days," more than a hundred times is crazy-making. But my friends' concerned acceptance of what I'm saying—over and over—has kept me from going crazy.

Tell stories about the outside world. My friends' tales of office dalliances, children's cheeky shenanigans, and the latest twist in a celebrity scandal have successfully distracted me from the isolation of the sick world for years. Even better has been real life in action, like when my next-door neighbor Maureen, or, as my sister calls her, my seventy-two-year-old roommate, stood over me as I lay in bed in a semi-hallucinogenic state of pain.

"Oh, you poor love," Maureen cooed while softly petting the top of my head. "Now, what do you think of my new red shoes?" She stood back a few feet from my mirror, twirled her ankle, and put her hand on her hip. "Aren't they very smart?" she asked, clearly delighted with the purchase. I used my remaining strength to lift up my head a few inches from the pillow. "They're lovely, Maureen. Really, lovely." As my head fell back down, I couldn't help but laugh at this otherworldly distraction.

Hold my hand. In my sickest and darkest hours, nothing feels better than when a friend takes my hand. This simple gesture demonstrates what great friendships can do: "To brush the gray out of your skies and leave them only blue."*

*from an Edgar Guest poem, "A Friend's Greeting"

Originally appeared in *The Huffington Post,* 2011

WHAT HELPED ME THROUGH

Green & Black's hot chocolate (four heaping teaspoons), hand holding, Arrested Development *Season One, friends with big ears, baby monitor (yes, it was for me), fantastically warm gloves, Xanax, velour sweatsuits in a rainbow of colors, Irish nurses. Anything funny—cards, YouTube videos, skits, and stories—it's hard to be scared when you're laughing. And always, always: family.*

SECONDHAND CANCER:
The Family of a Cancer Patient Is Sick, Too. They Just Don't Know It. Here's How to Heal.

Cindy Finch

As a hospital social worker, there's nothing quite like being "fired" by a patient's family. When it happened to me, I felt shocked and dismayed. When a comforting coworker saw the distress on my face and listened to my story, he said, "It's hard on families when someone they love has cancer. They all get knocked down by it."

He was right, and I learned a good lesson: a cancer diagnosis for one member of a family really means that the whole family gets sick. The hard part is that there is only one identified patient in the group. Everyone else just has to limp his or her way through it. But make no mistake, everyone is affected. When one member of the family is terminally or traumatically ill, they are all ill. They don't have cancer—they have what I call secondhand cancer.

Secondhand cancer is insidious. It makes people sick as much as secondhand smoke does: stealthily, without their quite being aware of it. There is no medicine for this illness. The depression, anger, exhaustion, grief, and anxiety of caregiving go largely unnoticed in many medical settings.

Caregivers, the dedicated friends and family members alongside their loved ones in the midst of a traumatic or terminal illness, are the ones most vulnerable to secondhand cancer. They're the people who stay when everybody else goes home. The "givers" hover over the beds of their loved ones or keep a serene vigil by their side while nurses, technicians, housekeepers, doctors, consultants, food trays, and other visitors file in and out of the room to care for the patient. They keep watch. They leave only to call home before they catch a quick nap in a waiting room chair.

Their love and sense of duty toward a sick or dying person have sucked the life out of them and left them virtually empty. They become patients in their own right—but no one seems to notice.

You know that caregiving has taken its toll when you see their pale faces in the room, or watch them break down when, after long days and nights of giving care, they are met by bad or worse news from the physician they thought was going to heal their loved one. When off duty and relieved by another giver, those closest to the patient often walk the halls of the hospital like zombies, exhausted by long stints in the room, depleted from talking to so many different people in a medical language unfamiliar to them, wasted from continually holding up the banner of hope to the sick one, burdened from all that has been and haunted by all that may still be.

Unlike the patient, caregivers have to deal with their illness alone. Their desperation and fear have to be dealt with privately, away from their loved one, because these valiant folks have to, at all costs, protect their beloved from their own needs and from the sadness they carry that no one can help them with. It would be a horrendous violation of the unspoken code of givers to burden their patient with any more burdens.

In the medical field, we often recommend that patients recovering from surgery take some time off from work, lighten their duties, and get lots of rest. The same is true for caregivers—except no one tells them. So I will.

First, those experiencing secondhand illness can take care of themselves by simply acknowledging that they have been affected as much, if not more, than the patient has. The patient has an entire medical team caring for her or him, but the giver does not.

Second, talk to a trusted family member, friends, or a counselor about your loved one's illness and its effect on you. A person who can listen and "hold" your story will lighten your load and help free you from the isolation of caregiving.

Third, pace yourself. The approach of slow and steady wins the race. Try to keep things normal. Go for a walk. Don't forget to recharge with a nap or a funny movie. You need some R&R from the combat zone. Even nurses who are professional caregivers take time off.

Finally, utilize the abundance of technology that is available to manage the cumbersome tasks that can weigh you down, such as giving medical updates to faraway family and coordinating volunteers who want to help. Reimagine *(www.reimagine.me.com)* — the company I work for, Caring Bridge *(www.caringbridge. org)*, Lotsa Helping Hands *(www.Lotsahelpinghands.com)*, and Take Them a Meal *(www.Takethemameal.com)* are just a few of the many websites dedicated to helping the families and friends — the givers — of someone who is sick.

Take advantage of these sources of help, and any others that come your way. Remember: the better you feel, the more you can help.

Originally appeared in *Reimagine* magazine, 2014, and *The Huffington Post*, 2014

MY ANGST LIST

Reading scriptures. Prayer. Laughter. Ice cream. My friends and family.

SHE IS HERE TO SING

Leslie Purchase

I knew it was cancer when I saw it on the ultrasound screen. Before I had three children—ages four, two, and six months, at that point—I was a surgeon. When I felt the lump, my husband made an appointment with a local breast surgeon. When she put the ultrasound probe on my breast and we saw calcifications, I knew in my heart what it meant. My husband, an orthopedic surgeon himself, was in absolute denial.

No one wants to consider his or her own mortality, and, in that moment, I remember thinking, so this is how I am going to die. The lump was big enough to feel. That, coupled with my young age, was not reassuring. When my sentinel node tested positive, it seemed likely that I would not survive this diagnosis. Darkness descended. Everything was fraught with emotion. Even buying new clothes seemed worthless. What was the point if I were only going to die soon anyway?

Looking back on these thoughts, now, is both painful and healing all at once. If I could speak to the me of that time, I would say, *Don't worry. It will be bad, but in the end you will be all right.* I cannot go back in time and say that to the terrified mother of three small children, but I can say that to you, the reader of this book. Those of us who have stood in that dark place and returned to tell the tale are obligated to share those stories of darkness and light, and the journeys we took between the two.

Olivia, my youngest daughter, was only six months old when I learned I had breast cancer. As I sit here typing my story, Olivia, now age six, is playing and singing at the top of her lungs. She has her own story of cancer, but that is for another time.

Back to my dark days. I won't bore you with the details of my tumor, but long story short, I endured some brutal treatment and, in the end, I am still here. That, in the end, is all you need to know about my experience with cancer, because, in the end, that is all that mattered to me. I am here listening to my daughter sing. She is here to sing. What else could I ask for?

There are battle scars. My breasts are no longer the ones I was born with. I don't have feeling in the back of my right arm. I had emergency surgery once, and planned surgery six more times. But all you need to know about me is that I am happy post-cancer.

There is still joy after cancer.

There is love after cancer.

In a word, there is life after cancer.

What matters most is that there is still life . . . even with cancer. And just like my daughter, I still get to sing.

WHAT HELPED ME STAY SANE

During my time wandering in cancer land, there were a surprising number of things that helped. I say surprising, because, when you are diagnosed, it is hard to imagine being able to feel comfort again. But, all is not lost. There is much joy, comfort, and love, even with cancer.

1. Cultivate laughter. Laughter is some truly wonderful medicine. Even though, when you are sick, it may be the farthest thing from your mind, it can do wonders for your body. I forced loved ones to watch funny movies or TV series with me. Consider having distant friends and relatives make videos of themselves telling jokes to send to you. Laughter lightens and is incredibly important. Let "there is humor in everything" become your new mantra.

2. Baby yourself. No rushing or stressing, to the extent that that is possible. Eat good food, take your time, read a good book, sip tea, and release expectations for yourself. It is the gift of time that is most in peril during your diagnosis. Give yourself permission to let go of everything that is not worth your time while you are in treatment.

3. Maintain a support system. We used the Caring Bridge site (www.caringbridge.org) to foster and organize our network of friends, loved ones, and acquaintances. It was therapeutic for me to write about my experiences, and it was a way to spread information without having to write it out or say it twenty times. Also, reading the guest responses always buoyed our spirits.

4. Ask for help. During the darkest days of my cancer and my daughter's cancer, I would reach out to our network for help. They are desperate to help. When I lost the ability to be grateful, I asked them to respond with what they were grateful for. When I lost the ability to see myself as beautiful, I asked them to respond with how they saw themselves as beautiful. When I lost the ability to be kind, I asked people to perform kindness in the world in our honor. Every time I asked, the response was incredibly inspiring and just what we needed to get over whatever heartache we were going through. The flip side of this is that everyone wants to help, even the people on the other side of the country. Everyone can be kind to someone or donate blood in your honor. Give people the gift of being useful.

My wish is that these suggestions bring some comfort to you during your sojourn in cancer land. See you on the other side . . .

Best,
Leslie

HOW TO BE YOUR OWN (BEST) MEDICAL RESEARCHER

Neil B. Feldman

I am a stage IV renal cancer patient. Many kinds of cancers, such as renal, might not cause symptoms to warn of the seriousness of the disease (or lead to early detection). Hearing the initial diagnosis can overwhelm the patient with shock and disbelief. I remember thinking, *Did I do something to cause this?*

It is a profound question worth considering with care.

The standard answer is that, perhaps aside from a few known risk factors (i.e., a history of smoking, exposure to toxic fumes, type 2 diabetes, or obesity), the cause of your cancer remains unknown. Many "old school" medical doctors and oncologists, when queried, will tell their patients, "There is nothing you did to cause this cancer, and there's nothing you can do to cure it. Only surgery or medication will be of any use." But is that statement, that "only surgery or medication will be of any use," totally accurate? Is there anything more we can do to help stop the progression or the development of metastases?

I feel that, in fact, there is something more that we can do— if we choose to undertake our own medical research and act on it (in consultation with our doctors, of course). First, we can look at the basics over which we do have control, such as diet, nutrition, and other lifestyle changes. Second, we can delve into the medical and scientific research to keep abreast of the latest exciting and potentially lifesaving discoveries. This can be done by cancer patients or by their caregivers.

Some oncologists plead ignorance on the subject of proper nutrition and diet. Maybe medical school did not train them in the field of nutrition. Or they are concerned that taking oral supplements may interfere with the metabolism of targeted or chemo drug therapies. This can create a confusing state of affairs for new patients who are left on their own, if they wish to become more proactive.

I am an advanced stage IV renal cancer patient who became convinced (alas, only after being diagnosed with bone metastases) that paying attention to proper diet and lifestyle changes might be of additional benefit to cancer patients and/or those hoping to avoid getting cancer in the first place.

By education and experience, I am an electrical engineer. My approach is to stay firmly grounded in science-based medicine (SBM) and evidence-based medicine.[1] In addition, I try to filter most of my research by always considering what standard medical care might look like twenty years in the future.

Thanks to the Internet, we now have the tools literally at hand to find, research, and most importantly, evaluate the full range of scientific opinions with relative ease. With so much data available at our fingertips, it may seem overwhelming to separate fact from fiction. But is that any reason to be timid when a very precious thing—your own life—is in peril?

To be a good researcher you must always have a healthy degree of skepticism toward what you read, even the peer-reviewed research published in reputable journals. Scientific knowledge, after all, is only as good as the questions posed and the experiments conducted. In this regard, I believe that anyone can become his or her own best medical researcher.

A good place to start is with the superb clearinghouse of medical research hosted by the National Institutes of Health and National Cancer Institute at PubMed *(www.ncbi.nlm.nih. gov/pubmed/)*. Papers published here by the NIH/NCI are usually free and complete. Others from universities, hospitals, and other scientific and medical establishments may only provide an abstract. They may require you to pay a fee to read or download the entire paper.

At first, reading these papers with their specialized nomenclature and medical language may feel like you're wandering into a foreign country without a guide or interpreter. Stay with it. Eventually, you will get accustomed to reading and even using this language. At the very least, this may impress or amuse your family and friends. Online resources such as Smart Patients *(www.SmartPatients.com)* and Wikipedia *(www.Wikipedia.org)* can help you get oriented and familiar with the terminology and acronyms rather quickly.

But now that you have your hands on the original research, how do you interpret the data? This is the hardest part. Here are some basic tips:

1. Observational studies cannot prove causation while random controlled trials can. In evaluating scientific data, and, in particular, conflicting or ambiguous opinions, one of the first things to consider is whether the conclusions are based on observational studies or the more rigorous random controlled trials (RCTs).

Observational studies can only serve to suggest hypotheses that can then be subjected to clinical studies (RCTs) that may or may not establish actual causation. This short video illustrates the distinction: *www.youtube.com/watch?v=UCk_yTkS6bU.*

2. Correlation does not prove causation. Beware of confounding factors that are overlooked or not acknowledged. For example, while observational studies a decade or so ago concluded that coffee drinkers had an increased risk of cancer, recent observational studies find, to the contrary, a reduced risk of cancer. Clearly, coffee alone is not the risk factor.

3. A finding of a "significant" result only means that the researcher feels that there is a greater than 95 percent assurance that the findings are not due to chance.

4. After studying the full paper, ask yourself, do the raw results actually support the author's/authors' conclusions?

5. Always search for the actual difference in the results, not the relative difference (expressed as a percentage). Relative changes often allow the results to look far more impressive than they actually are.

6. Many people are uncomfortable with statistics—with good reason. "The Median Isn't the Message," an essay by famed scientist Stephen Jay Gould, illustrates the problem well: *www.cancerguide.org/median_not_msg.html.* Gould was told his cancer would kill him, but he went on to live another twenty years.

These tips are by no means exhaustive. Keep in mind that whether you or another person in your familial or social circles takes on the task of doing the research, these same tips will still apply.

I often share the results of any new research with my oncologists, friends, family, and other caregivers. The fact is, it's almost impossible for busy doctors to keep up to date with all of the latest papers—especially cutting-edge research that has not made its way into the clinic quite yet. I have found that forward-thinking doctors and caregivers really appreciate such a "heads-up," and the discussions that often follow can be very informative.

Based on my own experience over the past year, I can say that researching my cancer and discussing my findings with doctors, family, and friends have let me play an active role in fighting my disease. I believe this has made me a better patient. It has also helped me maintain a certain sense of optimism and peace that also communicates some relief to my family and friends. Learning about what medical science understands about cancer today and what the prospects are for a lasting cure in the future buoy them.

I hope it buoys you, too.

THE ONE SPECIAL ITEM THAT GOT ME THROUGH THE NIGHTS

My constant research.

[1] Based on my research in scientific and medical journals, I have also experimented on myself. As a result, I have reached my own conclusions about the efficacy of various dietary suggestions made by "experts," government entities, and various medical associations. I have become appalled by what is commonly thought to be a "healthy" diet and stunned to realize that for over forty years so much bad nutritional advice has been advocated without any hard scientific proof. This has resulted in a giant "science project" perpetrated on the public for decades. The result has been a dramatic increase in levels of obesity, type 2 diabetes, and other examples of the "metabolic syndrome." All of these conditions have been associated with an increase in the risk of cancers and other deadly diseases.

NO CREDENTIALS REQUIRED:
Advocating for a Friend with Cancer
Holly Pruett

Ever since funeral directors offered to "undertake" whatever families couldn't handle, care for our beloved dying and dead has become the purview of professionals. These days, specialists function more like "partialists." For the newly diagnosed and those living with a terminal illness: Who keeps track of the big picture? Who helps navigate the whirling maze of doctors, pharmacies, clinical trials, treatment appointments, complementary care, and insurance coverage, not to mention basic household management?

It is easy to feel intimidated by the complexities of the medical-industrial complex; easy to feel defeated by a terminal or life-threatening diagnosis compounded by a seemingly endless array of needs.

That's why we, friends of those living with dying, need to step up. In 2010, my close friend Marcy Westerling was diagnosed, out of the blue, with stage IV ovarian cancer. I have been privileged to be by her side from the first bleak night after she received her diagnosis, alone in her car on the side of the highway. Her suffering saddens me deeply; the chance to "do something" to ease the way provides some measure of solace.

Of the various forms of support I've helped put in place (detailed below), what Marcy has valued the most is direct advocacy with the system to cut through its red tape and endless denials. In her words, she'd like to see more of us "stubbornly pushing and pushing and meeting all the insipid and occasionally useful demands of the system" to get our loved ones into the best trials and with the best providers. Taking on the calls and faxes and tracking, telling the back-story again and again, asking about things that seem off the table—what Marcy describes as "the things that would have overwhelmed me on my own and overwhelm most peer patients I know, as they settle for what is offered them versus what might benefit them more."

Here are some of the practices that have helped us, Marcy's close circle of friends, advocate on her behalf and walk with her into Cancer World.

1. *Assemble a Health Profile*—Chances are, a second opinion is in order, as well as the application forms for clinical trials, and the access information for any number of other providers. As a friend, you can help by pulling all of the information together into a single document. This health profile should include the person's date of birth, spouse, contact information, and insurance policy numbers; the diagnosis (using specific clinical language); details of all treatments to date; results of all tests; and contact information for all members of the health care team. Once assembled, this document should be kept up to date and furnished to any new or prospective members of the health care team.

2. *Wrangle Red Tape* — The search for optimal treatment may include switching among a myriad of specialists. This will necessitate record transfers, determination of eligibility, scheduling of appointments. With a signed release of information, designating you as a friend/medical advocate, you can make these calls and order these record transfers on behalf of the patient.

3. *Set Up a Communications System* — Receiving the well-wishes of a large community of concerned people can be as burdensome as it is comforting for those who are seriously ill. It's hard enough to keep one's own head above water. Loved ones have needs, especially around feelings of helplessness, grief, and loss. Someone should step up to talk to them. It is not the patient's job to assuage their pain. At the same time, if the person's community is to support the patient through sickness and even dying, that same community needs care and feeding. As a friend, you can attend to the needs of the broader community by setting up a communications platform like Caring Bridge. This enables updates to reach a broad number of people, and for those folks to post their love and prayers without expectations of a response.

4. *Coordinate Support* — Your loved one may need meals cooked, errands done, rides provided. An online tool like Lotsa Helping Hands can streamline messages about what the needs are, providing automated reminders for those who sign up to take care of specific tasks.

5. *Research Options* — Are there clinical trials that should be considered? Other providers who might be a better fit? Services

that could ease some of the burdens related to treatment, like housing and transportation? As a friend, you can take on these research tasks, using the Internet and the phone to track down answers.

6. *Provide Eyes and Ears*—No patient should go to a doctor's appointment alone. The company of a spouse or family member may be comforting, but that person may be too caught up in his or her own secondary trauma to listen well or take good notes. As a friend, you can help by discussing in advance the goals for the appointment, bringing a written copy of all questions, writing down every word of what is said in the appointment (alternately, asking the doctor's permission to record it with a smartphone), paraphrasing back all key points to the doctor or care provider to confirm understanding, and then writing up a summary of the appointment afterwards.

Doctors, social workers, counselors, nutritionists, acupuncturists, chaplains—all of these professionals with impressive initials after their names have vital roles to play. Equally important, though, is the role of medical companion—the friend who shows up and helps to carry some small portion of the load.

The skills required are no more than basic organization, the ability to follow through, and respect for the wishes of the one who is ill. For those things you don't know how to do, such as using some of the online research or communication tools, you can recruit someone who does. The most durable support is provided by a team, with one or two people acting as team leaders to coordinate the division of labor.

The tasks described here can be time consuming, but the

rewards are invaluable. From helpless to helpful; from despairing to engaged; from isolated to connected—acting in support of your sick or dying friend is time you will never regret spending. Walking by Marcy's side since her diagnosis has taught me so much about life, death, friendship, and myself.

For those who are ill, may you have friends to companion your every step.

WHAT GETS ME THROUGH THE ANGST OF CANCER

1. *Being active: doing what I can to ease the suffering of those living with cancer.*

2. *Remembering well: honoring the memory and legacy of those who have died, keeping them alive in the world through valuing all that their lives and deaths nourished.*

3. *Getting ready: learning everything I can about living with and dying of cancer, and how to grieve the sickness and death of loved ones, to become more skillful at living with a heart broken open by it all.*

NANCY NOVACK IS MY HEROINE

Linda Novack

She also happens to be my sister. I really didn't want to write this and have to relive all the painful times surrounding my sister Nancy's cancer. But the other side pulled harder. There is so much to share to bring hope and inspiration to others on their journeys. And I want you to know how the "A Team" played an integral part in Nancy's journey.

This all started over ten years ago. One day, before I was leaving for a vacation to France, I received a call from my cousin Leslie that sent excruciating shock waves through my whole system. Nancy was at Stanford Hospital and had just been diagnosed with stage IV ovarian cancer, and it had already metastasized into her liver. *What! How can this be? It can't be true.* But true it was. After reeling for a few hours, there was no question as to what I needed to do. I cancelled my trip to France, and the next day—or was it the same day?—I got into my car and drove up to Palo Alto.

Upon arrival at the hospital, I found my sister in a room receiving loving support from our cousin Leslie. Though Leslie and I stared at each other, devastated, trying to hide our fears and tears right there, we planted the roots of Nancy's A Team.

We had to be present and be there: while doctors determined the course of treatment for Nancy; through more chemo and more chemo and more chemo; during healing from the treatments; and even during trips, as all of us drove up and down the coast to help. The A Team consisted of close family and friends, bonded together in determination and commitment to Nancy's healing and ultimate wellness. We would sit and sometimes lie around her bed, while she was recovering from chemo, and laugh, yes laugh. It was all too heavy not to lighten it up. And Nancy would say, "I don't really have cancer!" And we would heartily agree. We would go shopping for wigs at the local Marin wig store watching Nancy transform herself into Marilyn Monroe with the sexy blond wigs, and then into someone who looked eerily like me in the red wigs. We would take Nancy to her chemo treatments and read healing visualizations while she sat there soaking in the "medicine." People would deliver delicious dinners, and we would cook.

We never let that diagnosis of stage IV ovarian cancer, and what that might mean, run our minds. As her A Team, we never bought into it. (As individuals late at night, yes, the scary, horrible thoughts crept in.)

And then there was Nancy's Doctor Brandy, the amazing angel who was brought to Nancy to guide her every medical choice with such precision and confidence and kindness and commitment to her getting well. Truly, this doctor was the biggest A in the A Team. A Team, we came to know, meant Angels Team.

And there were so many other angels who miraculously came in to heal in their own special, unique ways. The village kept growing.

You really never know where your angels are going to come from, or when another one will show up on your doorstep. But they did and they do, and that's one of the little secrets that most doctors don't tell you. There will be the very dark and terrifying times and, side by side, an angel will appear out of the darkness bringing the Light back into the room.

Never underestimate the power of your very special angels to show up for you when you need them most.

And by the way, the Light won out, and Nancy is well and happy and kicking up a storm ten years after her diagnosis!

WHAT HELPED ME MOST

So many things helped me through my sister's cancer: meditation, reading inspirational books, prayers, visualizations, and finally understanding that her health was out of my control. I could support and love her in all sorts of ways, but ultimately I didn't have the power to save her. I could only hold the faith and the vision that she would be fine, one way or another. And then I learned to let go and allow, rather than trying to control.

BEING PRESENT
Leslie Roth

Though the events of Nancy Novack's illness have been indelibly, visually engraved in my memory, this written reiteration is most difficult.

I am the person, the cousin, who sat with Nancy as she received the bad news. And I am the person who had to relay the bad news to those who became her "A Team."

We had been discussing the logistics of driving to Los Angeles together, when Nancy disclosed a physical condition that sounded like classic appendicitis to my physician husband and me. I insisted she see a doctor before we traveled, which she did the next morning.

When her play-by-play reports from the driving, parking, and arrival at the office, just a few blocks from my home, stopped, I decided to walk over to the building, picking up magazines and snacks along the way, sure that I would be waiting for her outside of the operating room. I found her in the hospital's imaging area where we were directed to go immediately to her doctor's office.

The bad news, stage IV ovarian cancer, knocked us off our chairs. A flurry of emotional and logistical activity conducted us into a new world, all happening so quickly that we barely had time to hang onto our hugs and tears. In spite of the shock and the apparent urgency created in our midst, we somehow took care of business. We called Linda, Nancy's sister, and immediately ran back to my house to gather ourselves in preparation for the wild ride ahead. It was that urgent. No going back home, Nancy. Go directly to Stanford. How did we ever stay on the road? How did we enter a hospital that, when we finally arrived, we had no idea where to go? How did this part run as smoothly as it did? Or did it? We were in such an altered state and yet, somehow, we were being taken care of, gently integrated into the world of Cancer.

After the first shock of paperwork in admissions, where I was signed on as the person to make decisions for Nancy (in the case that she would not be able to?!), the next most alarming moment came as we walked into the unit with the sign over the doors, claiming this unrecognizable place to be the Cancer Center. Numbness. We clung to each other and entered. As Nancy prepared herself to be a patient and hopped into the hospital bed, her question to me, the first of many to follow over the next year, was, "Am I going to die?" And thus began my own personal dance with death as I tried to answer with honesty and hope, assurance but fear, authority fueled by love and complete ignorance.

We waited. We waited for a team of doctors and nurses who streamed in throughout the evening, with their questions and declarations and tests. And finally the doctor who was assigned to save Nancy's precarious life arrived, delivering the touch and the words that she would never forget, his promise to stay with her: "I am with you."

My job was to hold her hand and to contact her grown son and close friends. It was nighttime. My husband Bob had arrived after his workday at a San Francisco hospital. After a day of extreme emotional intensity, I had to leave Nancy and return home, hoping she could get some sleep; hoping I could, too.

The next day would begin the induction into a process none of us had ever expected to experience. With the arrival of Nancy's son Steven and her sister Linda, we began to form, without an utterance of acknowledgment, what would become a core support group — the team that, without question, would be with her throughout the term of her battle. The drivers, the hand holders, the entertainers, the midnight phone conversationalists, the unwavering crew who were not going to leave her alone. Never alone. Somehow, even with her disbelief that she actually had cancer, she knew it was worth all the pain and discomfort, all the scary nights and days, and all the frightening news that came her way, to fight for her life. Somehow it became apparent that, despite the gravity of the situation, it would be humor that kept Nancy and her A Team going. And when she asked, on occasion, if she were going to "make it," my dance would go into action again.

I searched for more reasons to tell her to hang in there; I was given some words of wisdom and a good book to read on hope — *The Anatomy of Hope: How People Prevail in the Face of Illness* by an oncologist, Dr. Jerome Groopman. He questioned how some patients continued on and on with the devastating treatments. He found that those who did were able to withstand the overwhelming side effects, all the while, with the belief that if they could stay alive, there was hope for new medical discoveries and innovations that might come along to make them whole again.

It was this small bit of information that gave me fortitude and focus to be strong for Nancy and to impart to her words of hope. She displayed a sense of inner strength that was previously unknown. She was not alone. I think she concentrated on hope and life. And she made it!

Being a caregiver for a cancer patient is a difficult task. I cannot say that it is possible for everyone to do the job well. It takes a lot of intuitiveness, something that may or may not come easily. If you have the time and can do it well, lucky you and lucky recipient. If you don't, perhaps you can contribute your own brand of support, and, along with the support of others, help create a team of effective caregivers.

I personally find it a natural state to watch closely and read someone's needs. I sat with my ailing mother, cooked for her, listened to her as she listed her wishes, played with my young child at her feet, held her hand. I lay on the bed with my cousin, who had breast cancer, and chatted about all the family stories that she loved to remember. I walked with my girlfriend and helped bathe her and prepare food for her. And I sat with my husband day and night, watched for his every need, bathed him and kept his surroundings just as he wished with his kids near him.

Whatever you do, you must do it without questions. You need to read the fear and anxiety and pain on your person's face and body before she or he can even tell you. Sometimes people want to be silent, and you will just have to be in the room, present but not intrusive. Always listen when they express their fears and doubts: never tell them they must not think those thoughts or suppress them. You can talk of hope, but, when there appears to be no happy ending, don't deny them the ability to say their goodbyes, either. Reading another person's needs takes concentration and watching. I clearly remember carefully moving Nancy into seating positions in hospital waiting rooms to keep her as comfortable as possible in very stressful times.

An important part of support is being the other perspective and the other ear. Try to hear the medical professionals and remember what they say, by taking notes, because it can be overwhelming for the patient. You can offer additional information to the physician about your loved one's mental and physical condition. You are the interviewer and the reporter.

The sum of your duties is to be present. Be there fully. Whether you offer a better seating position, or a fresh, cool drink, or you read a story aloud, or play favorite music, keep the comfort of your loved one at the heart of your intention.

HOW TO WOO A DOCTOR
Aisling Carroll

I drive past my HMO's "increase your laugh expectancy" bulletin board. I swear and stare down at chaotic pages of doctors' reports, which teeter across the hand brake of my car. As I jerk my head back up to the freeway in front of me, I recite phrases from the reports aloud. I give myself extra points if I correctly match the doctor to the phrase. This is my pre-appointment prep.

Thirty minutes later, I crisscross the patient parking lot while I clip in my fake pearl earrings. Today, I meet a new doctor, and I want her to know she's dealing with a professional patient who needs and respects her. And who will do just about anything to woo her.

After more than six years of, "This young woman presents with . . . rare . . . unusual . . . fascinating," I have seen at least a dozen doctors in hospitals and medical offices around the world. Doctors who helped send my ovarian cancer into remission, and others who now try to unravel why my pre-cancer health has not been restored.

Wanting to be that special patient who crowds the doctor's thoughts, I engage in everything from mild flirtation to outrageous baking. Then I pit doctor against doctor, hoping to appeal to their competitive streak. I am also not below addressing them by title, in every sentence, nor branding my collection of symptoms a "House" case, which is theirs to famously crack.

Below are the top five things I know about doctors:

1. The calmer the doctor, and the closer she sits, the worse the news. Recovering from surgery for a burst cyst, I sat in my hospital bed and giddily studied the Irish newspaper ad for "Sunway Travel! Canary Islands—seven nights, self-catering! Sale starts today!" when my doctor quietly walked in, put her clipboard down and pulled up a chair. Until then, she had been a hurricane of manila files and beeps, talking to me with one foot in the hallway and one in my room. As a result, her newfound attention was flattering. Maybe my efforts at good hospital cheer were paying off? Maybe she wanted to chat about the new Ian McEwan novel she spotted earlier next to my bedside? And maybe, the best possible scenario, she was about to grant my request to be released early? But that winter's day, sitting less than thirty-six inches across from me, she told me I had ovarian cancer. Almost two years later, when another busy doctor walked into my narrow, gray room, sat by my side, and acted as if he had all the time in the world, I knew instantly: "I'm screwed."

2. Never use the verb "google." Google a new medical term, pop a Xanax, write the information on a flashcard. (Repeat.) In the first few weeks of my diagnosis, this was my night's work when everyone else had gone to bed. So by the time my second meeting with my oncologist rolled around, I didn't feel too poorly

prepared, but my jaw was becoming increasingly locked, and I could feel my heart beating in my head. When the doctor walked into the examination room, we exchanged handshakes, short smiles, and lamentations about the rain. Then I said: "When I googled clear cell carcinomas on www.cancercures. com the other night . . ." and he heard, "www.my-doctor-don't-know-s**t.com," the genial mood was ruined. Today, I still google; I just don't cop to it in front of the boss.

3. Swap the "patient as warrior" routine for a little vulnerability. Losing consciousness while dressed in combat trousers—five pockets and eight zippers per leg—the nurses wheeled me out of the chemo ward and into a side room. They wanted the doctor to see me. And I wanted him to see my warrior spirit. Attempting to smile with eyes shut, I led him to the conclusion I was tough enough. He smiled back, walked away, and I was left with nothing to stop my body's free fall. No new plan of attack. No new drugs. No new words of encouragement. I never made this mistake again. Months later, when my body was failing, I didn't act tough, but I also didn't act on my desperate desire to handcuff myself to the doctor, either. Instead, I held my hands together over my peach velour sweatpants and asked for his help.

4. Silence the note taker. Early on, I noticed that some doctors weren't so thrilled to have to answer additional questions from my note taker (read: my mom), as well as me. Sure, there was the one doctor who enjoyed an audience, but in my experience, most prefer a more intimate, one-to-one conversation. As a result, I now ask my mom to give me her questions in advance so she won't have to ask the doctor. Then when we walk into the

examination room, I banish her to the dodgy stool in the corner, out of the doctor's line of vision. I make up for this shoddy treatment with a trip to IHOP on our way home.

5. In crisis, always utter eight magical words. The once-off consultation with Dr. Conroy started out well. "You certainly have very good reflexes," he said, after hammering on my knee. "Oh, yes. Well, I've been working on that," I replied with a wince, instantly realizing how bad that lame flirtation sounded. Even worse, it didn't work. "I don't think there's anything else I can add here," he said as he closed my file and stood up. I tried to hide my shock and threw my eight-worded Hail Mary pass: "If you were me, what would you do?" He sat down and reopened the file.

The last thing I know about doctors is that the best ones have gone to the ends of the earth to keep me on it. Their Thanksgiving cards are in the mail.

Originally appeared in *The Huffington Post*, 2011

WHAT IS COURAGE?

"Cancer is just a bully.
Kick its ass so bad
it will never come back."
—Stand Up to Cancer

BIGGER THAN PRINCE

Bonnie Powers

Facing cancer is scary. In my immediate family alone, eight cancers have been diagnosed, my own melanoma included, and three of my four siblings carry the BRCA2 mutation. Witnessing cancer's ravages, most especially with my mother who lost her battle, I don't take the threat or diagnosis lightly. I know that rising above fear takes great courage, especially when hope is elusive.

To prepare for and recover mentally and physically from my recent prophylactic surgeries, I called up all the positive life force energy I could muster. Rather than falling into the trap of self-pity, I attempted to bring forth an indomitable spirit and brightness.

Trauma can be a very lonely place. The love of family and outpouring of support from so many near and far have lifted me on tough days and helped cheerlead me through the adversity. But trauma is also quite isolating, because no one but you can create the necessary functions for healing.

Cancer has shown me that there is no time to waste on anything but love and happiness. Yes, happiness. It's not always easy. Like any new skill, the more you do it, the better at it you become. When things get challenging, I remind myself of my very own indomitable spirit and brightness. And when it gets really tough, I put on my headphones, get my groove on, and "walk around like I'm bigger than Prince."

Originally appeared on Bonnie's website BRCA2: In This Together
www.brca2gether.wordpress.com

MY RESOURCES

What I read—
- *Positive Results* book
- *Positive Results* blog (*www.positiveresultsthebook.blogspot.com*)
- *Ticking Time Bombs* blog (*www.tickingtimebombsblog.com*)
- *Me, Redone* blog (*www.meredone.com/category/brca/*)
- *The Pink Moon Lovelies: Empowering Stories of Survival* book
- *F Cancer website—Education on Early Detection*
  (*www.letsfcancer.com*)
- *Anticancer: A New Way of Life* book
- *Anticancer: A New Way of Life* website (*www.anticancerbook.com*)
- *Healthy Child Healthy World: Creating a Cleaner, Greener,*
  Safer Home book
- *Healthy Child Healthy World* website (*www.healthychild.org*)

Support Groups—
- *FORCE, Facing Our Risk of Cancer Empowered*
- *BRCA Sisterhood Closed Facebook Group*
- *Bright Pink*

Pre-surgery tips for double mastectomy—
- *Two weeks prior, wean off caffeine. You want the blood flow to*
all of your blood vessels to be as optimal as possible.

• *Prepare for your welcome home by putting things you'll use regularly at table height. You won't be able to reach up for anything for a few weeks. You may not even have the strength to open the refrigerator door, so plan for this in advance.*

• *Make sure any medications are in non-child-proof bottles. You won't likely have the strength to open them.*

• *Sit in the back seat of the car on the way home from the hospital. If there were an accident, you don't want to be hit with air bags from the front.*

• *Change your voicemail with updates so that you don't have to spend energy you won't have those first days/weeks talking, and repeating how you are doing.*

• *Limit visits and don't feel the need to prep for visits or entertain anyone. This is about your healing and reserving your energy to do just that.*

• *When you are cleared to shower, know that you can't get the drain sites wet (moisture = bacteria). Loop your drains around your neck and use big safety pins to attach them (to what, I'm not sure yet!).*

• *Do not apply lotion, deodorant, or perfume near your incisions.*

Mastectomy resources —

• *Post mastectomy, Breast Comfort Pillows work well for the car ride home to protect your sides, incisions, and sore muscles, and while you are at home on the computer or in bed. I met Shirley, a cancer survivor, mom, and the founder of Precious Survivors, at an event with her daughter, Rachel, a BRCA2 previvor and author of* Ticking Time Bombs. *Shirley hand-makes these little heart-shaped pillows.*

• *Extra king-sized pillows to prop up in bed and use for side*

140

support. *I understand that I won't have the muscle strength to get up from a flat lying position, and we do not have a recliner, so we bought some extra-full king-sized pillows at Marshalls, so I can sleep propped up. I'll probably also add a neck pillow.*

• Straws: *If you have tightness in your chest and find it hard to take deep breaths after surgery, breathing through a straw is supposed to help. We bought metal straws at a bar supplies store.*

• Caution: *If you are considering using a heating pad on your stomach, if you are suffering from constipation, note that you do not want the heating pad near your breasts/wounds. You won't have sensation there and you could get burned without realizing it (your skin is very sensitive from the surgery).*

What's on my bedside table —
• *Steel water bottle*
• *Second chakra aromatherapy spray*
• *Ricolas*
• *Organic vanilla rosemary lip balm*
• *Olbas natural inhaler to open nasal passages with a refreshing cooling feeling*
• *Bell (gift from a colleague; Jeff had a chuckle)*
• *Blum Naturals organic chamomile natural cloth face wipes*
• *Honest plant-based natural cloth body wipes*
• *Cucumber cool face toner spray*
• *Tea Tree and Lavender deodorant*
• *Bach Rescue Pastilles for natural stress relief*
• *Origins "Peace of Mind" on-the-spot relief*
• *Arnica gel*
• *Aleve*
• *Colace*

DANCING WITH THE NICE COWBOY

Gabrielle Roth

Waves move in patterns. Patterns move in rhythms. A human being is just that—energy, waves, patterns, rhythms. Nothing more. Nothing less. A dance.

May I have the courage to live through all the things that my life dance reveals to me. All the things I've pushed down inside that need to come up and out through me, so I can be an empty vessel of perfection, of love.

May I have the courage to get out of my way, to become all that I am, and to hook myself up with my deepest yearnings. To stand up for my truth. To break through my own walls of resistance.

May I have the courage to embrace my body while it's still here. To express my heart. To allow it to be part of my body, part of my spontaneity, part of my expression.

May I have the courage to let my head go and trust that there is something guiding me. That there is some enormous amazing purpose to my existence. That I wasn't thrown here as some accidental afterthought of some mean cowboy.

May I have the courage to stand with my own story, what ever it is and was. To know that I and only I have the power to erase it and to move beyond its confines, however good, or bad, or weird, or twisted, or wondrous they may have been. They were and I am.

May I have the courage to witness another, to encourage, to celebrate, to support, to catalyze their growth, to be committed to the poetry of their existence.

May I have the courage to be myself. To be real. And may I please have the courage to stand up for those who cannot stand up for themselves.

FEAR

Alexander Niles

What is fear?

I read that fear is an emotional response induced by a perceived threat, which causes a change in brain and organ function, as well as in behavior. Fear can lead us to hide, to run away, or to freeze in our shoes. Fear may arise from a confrontation, or from avoiding a threat, or it may come in the form of a discovery.

When I was younger, fear came in the form of a scary movie, like *The Shining* or *Nightmare on Elm Street*. A little bit later, the fright was whether or not I would get picked in the neighborhood basketball game, and a little bit after that, it was which girl I should ask to the school dance. After that, dread was dealt in the form of finding a job after college, and then consternation came about keeping that same job.

The day I found out what true fear genuinely feels like came later, at age thirty. It didn't come in the form of a movie, or a girl. It came in the form of being diagnosed with stage IV cancer. It rushed into my life like a tsunami, reaping havoc and filling my mind with doubt and anxiety, my intellect with worry and the unknown. I was quite literally in fear of losing my life.

My first reaction was utter shock. I didn't know what was to come, but hearing words like cancer took the air out of me, as if I were punched in the gut by a heavyweight boxer. I knew that the fear I was experiencing was rational, and was certainly modulated by the process of cognition and learning. All the negative connotations with such an illness, and such a severe stage as well. Fear felt natural. It felt real. Ironically, it made me feel alive.

Clearly fear has a place in our lives, but I wasn't about to let it control me. No way would I allow it to dictate how I chose to live. Not a chance. It's easy to ignore our fears, but courage won't make it to the playing field unless you have a fear to face down. By owning my feelings, I took the first step toward gaining control over the situation as best I could.

Instead of ignoring the situation I found myself in, or denying its seriousness, I decided to address it head on. As the days and weeks passed, after hearing that dreadful diagnosis, I let that fear keep simmering. I acknowledged it, and began to keep a journal. At first, my diary served as a concession to panic, and slowly evolved into a way I would conquer it. I often look back on my journal during those early days, and it now serves to give me strength and encouragement, and also to see the big picture. It enabled me to track my progress as I worked towards conquering my fear.

After accepting and admitting my fear, I tried to chase negative thoughts from my mind—to picture what it would be like to win this battle, with a big wide smile on my face. I set that as my big goal, but also focused on smaller concrete goals to help me get there. I made it a point to meditate every day when I woke up, thinking about peaceful settings such as the wind blowing through a forest of healthy, green leaves on sturdy, deep-rooted trees. I imagined that I was lying on the forest floor, watching the limbs sway back and forth as I breathed in healing air, and breathed out unneeded thoughts or feelings.

Although it was paramount to commit to one outcome—overcoming my fear—I found it necessary to let myself be afraid at times. I realized there was no way to eliminate fear from my life entirely, and that this valid emotion was one that would build character, and teach me what I had within me, and how to act with courage.

Sometimes through the darkest skies, the brightest stars reveal themselves and shine. Although I never asked to be in this situation, being confronted by the darkest of fears, and accepting, confronting, and overcoming that fear enabled me to learn, grow, and be even more mortal. Feeling fear is human, but I assure you, conquering it will make you feel empowered, courageous, and proud.

Originally appeared in *Psychology Today*
and *The Huffington Post*, 2014

WHAT HELPED ME THROUGH

What helped me was taking a step back and identifying sources of anxiety in my life, and eliminating them one by one, so I could focus my efforts and energy on healing.

FIGHTING TERMINAL CANCER WITH LIFE

Lisa Marie Wilson

My mom had terminal cancer, and she fought until her last breath to beat it. She had a rare ocular melanoma that metastasized to her liver. For that type of melanoma, only 5 percent of patients will have tumor shrinkage using the chemo cocktails that are available in this day and age, because melanoma is pretty much unstoppable once it spreads. My mom knew the odds and went through a lot of pain to have a few more days of pain. I wish that I knew what I know now, and I had talked her out of chemo and into Hawaii.

No one wants to lose to cancer. Her doctor was the best we could have had, because he never treated her like she was dying. That's what she needed. If my cancer, that I have beaten so far, metastasizes, and I only have a 5 percent chance of adding a few months to my life, I am going to Hawaii. The debilitating pain that my mom endured with three rounds of full-body chemo and two infusions into her liver was horrible for her spirit. She wasn't even herself in the last few weeks because of the morphine pills.

Doctors are taught to save people. Period. As patients, we need to be realistic about what we actually need saving from. Do months of sickness in hopes of a miracle outweigh a peaceful, beautiful time spent with family and friends and love? When my mom got sick from chemo and lost her hair, she didn't want anyone to see her. So she pushed everyone away and didn't want visitors. It was the very opposite of what she needed in her last months on Earth.

If doctors were realistic to their terminal patients and said, "This isn't a cure. It's treatment to add time to your life, to hopefully slow down the tumors, but it won't stop them forever," would that change the fight? Fighting cancer is the hope of winning life. Doctors join our side of the fight with chemo, radiation, surgeries,` and drugs. When the fight is futile, and the odds are against us, our fight should be to experience the beauty of life. I'm not suggesting people give up on the fight; I'm only suggesting that you have to realize what you are actually fighting.

If you are fighting a cancer which always wins, is it worth losing the little life you have left? Becoming so sick that you stop enjoying the life around you is not really living at all. When loved ones decide, "No more treatment, I can't do it anymore," it's not giving up on life. It is living for the life they have left. We will be angry that they are leaving us. We will be sad to lose the relationship we had with them. We will bargain that if they try a little harder, they can win. We will deny that any of the cancer is happening but, in the end, we will accept that with life comes dying. We know that it's our fate from the first time we lose someone we love. Death is birth in reverse — we go back to which we came.

Everyone has to make the right choice for himself or herself. I made some decisions for my mom that I regret, because I was making them for my own selfish reason of not wanting to lose her. Each generation of my family has helped a parent deal with cancer and then gotten cancer themselves. My grandmother begged her father to fight harder to beat colon cancer, and he quit the fight of cancer and fought for what life he had left. At that moment, she vowed that if she ever got cancer, she would win, and she beat breast cancer. Sometimes terminal cancer patients do win against cancer, and I'm so grateful that miracles do happen. All I know is that for me, if I ever get the unfortunate news that I only have a 5 percent chance of living a few extra months, you will find me chemo-free on a beach. It will be the first time I won't be worrying about melanoma for myself, but I'll make sure my daughter is covered in sunblock.

Originally appeared in *The Huffington Post*, 2014

WHAT MADE MY HEALING HAPPEN

What helped me during my cancer journey was to find the humor in anything I could. I had just laughed with my mom while she fought terminal cancer, and then, post-mortem, she made me laugh as I kept her voice alive in my head. I did acupuncture for the pain. And I prepared everything I could in advance to make sure I had the food and pills I would need while I was super tired and sick. The main thing that kept me going was my daughter Amelia, as I didn't want to miss out on a minute of her life and our future together.

We can't stop cancer from taking lives, but we can stop cancer from taking the life inside us while we fight it with laughter, love, and hope.

DIVATUDE: Beauty in Spite of a Diagnosis

Daphne D. Evans

As a woman of curves, who believes in Walt Whitman's "female form divine," I had finally learned to embrace the dip and sway of my body—the pure sensuality of being a woman. I spent my childhood as "the fat girl," and my teen years battling anorexia. I weight-trained my way into womanhood, and just when I reached the best shape of my life, my doctor's words changed everything: "I regret to tell you, but you have been diagnosed with ovarian cancer." I was thirty-five.

I longed to have a child. The idea of losing a major part of my womanhood plunged me into despair. I had the surgery and became a career woman overachiever. I dropped down to a size three, having lost so much weight with the cancer, and felt I was at my most attractive, because I was finally thin. But as I look back, I see I was sick with body dysmorphia.

Seven years later, a mammogram showed a mass on my left breast. The ovarian cancer had metastasized—this news brought me to my knees. After a double mastectomy, I remember it clearly: I came home that day by myself, bandaged so tightly that my DDD chest was now flat as a board. I could not get past the mirrored armoire in the hallway. I stood there for countless minutes sobbing. I couldn't look myself in the eyes. Angry and depressed, I asked God, "Why is this happening to me? Don't you think I've gone through enough?"

But the next day, I awoke with this peace of quiet resolve, and the simple question *What I am going to do about this?* What would make me feel womanly again—full of sensuality and joie de vivre? I always loved going to spa. So I went that day and received massage treatments. Well, it was so wonderful that I went for an entire week! That's when I made a choice:

I will not let cancer define me or allow it to rob me of feeling beautiful and creating joyous experiences.

I began to dress more stylishly—stilettos became my friend. I had regular appointments to get my hair and nails done and even went to get eyelash extensions when mine began to fall out. I bought higher-count linens for my bed; spritzed them down with English lavender linen water before bedtime. One day I went to a high-end shop and bought all black lace lingerie! My gowns I wore for bed were 1930s vintage that I found on eBay—sensual and silky to the touch. I finally learned to put myself at the top of my priority list. I even coined a word for my new perspective: Divatude.

This beautiful Diva's story does not end there. In 2009, I was diagnosed with a third form of cancer: spinal. Right now, I thank God that all of my cancers are in remission. My message to my sisters is this: Yes, you have cancer. Your head is bald from the chemo, and you feel sick a lot of the time. But when you're what I call a Cancer Diva, you don't have to take any of it lying down. There's still so much to celebrate—starting with the fact that you're here.

In closing, I want you to know that I have helped so many women going through cancer maintain their inner fortitude and self-esteem through spa treatments. For us, beauty does count. Many women dealing with breast cancer have such a hard time with the mastectomy side of it. Quite a few of these ladies are like me, who had "big beautiful ones," and the identity crisis is hitting them hard. I decided to write a poem about our struggle.

THE BREASTPLATE OF BEAUTY

You look down,
Curves so familiar, so comforting,
They started young, got you noticed,
Blushing when the boys pointed,
Pulling out your sweater to try to hide them.
But they were yours and they were beautiful,
They were a part of you.
They grew with you,
Drove you crazy when trying to contain them,
Stretching your aching back when you carried them,
But you would give them up for nothing.
They were a part of you.
You dreamed of motherhood,
Again looking down,
Seeing the peaceful face of a child
Sweet, innocent tulip mouth in the natural state of supping.
Smiling, you held them close to you,
Wonderful nurturer that you are.
But now you must say good-bye with tears in your eyes,
Saying "farewell" to the gifts God has bestowed on every woman.

They did not define you as a person, but
They were a part of you.
Look up, woman warrior!
Let your battle scars become your breastplate of beauty,
Learn to stand tall again, straighten those shoulders that
    once held the weight,
A weight that is no longer there.
Look at yourself in the mirror,
And say, I am a beautiful warrior!
I have survived the battle and have overcome the war.
For though they are gone, I am alive!
And though they were a part of me,
I
AM
STILL
ME.

Copyright ©2013

THINGS THAT REALLY HELPED ME
GET THROUGH THE AGONIES OF CANCER

As head of Heaven's Door Cancer Foundation and a cancer survivor, I have firsthand experience in what inspires cancer patients and helps them through such a difficult time.

1. My faith in God comes head on the list. From going through tortuous spinal cancer and being bedridden for months in 2009-2010, my faith was renewed that I was not alone. Prayer and meditation are the keys to remaining strong.

2. Secondly, staying positive to help other cancer patients during my own struggle was important. During my spinal cancer, I had an old colonial house renovated by students from a local university. Though I was in bed at times, I created a "Healing Home" for women to come to and have massages and tea, to try on wigs, laugh, and share fellowship with each other.

3. Lastly, it is very important to take care of one's mental health and surround yourself with support and friends. During this last battle, there were times of loneliness. Depression, coupled with pain, feeds thoughts of suicide. I went through a suicide attempt. I now counsel others who are dealing with such problems. Without the help and prayers of friends and family, it would have been too much to bear.

Also taking time out to do something random just for one's self is important—shopping, going for a massage or a manicure, having date night with a spouse or partner, or a "buddy" night of going to listen to music, or something fun with friends.

My motto is this: Do not allow yourself to be defined by your cancer, no matter what stage you are in.

As Dylan Thomas says, "Do not go gentle in that good night . . . rage, rage against the dying of the light."

154

ONE ALMIGHTY EFFORT

Kevin Haugh

> "When the world says, 'Give up,' Hope whispers,
> 'Try it one more time.'" —Anonymous

I was born in the West Clare Peninsula on Ireland's Wild
Atlantic Way in 1954, and I spent my professional life teaching
in the Galvone-Southill inner-city community in Limerick
City, Ireland, from 1975 to my retirement in 2010. When I was
diagnosed with cancer in 2004, I was overwhelmed with the
support and goodwill that was showered upon my family and
me by people in both communities and especially those who
scarcely knew us.

Goodwill came to us in many forms and gave us the energy
to carry on. Equally, the divine powers people called upon,
especially Padre Pio and St. Matthew, to intervene on my behalf
delivered results in due course. I felt a noticeable turn for the
better in my battle with cancer around the time that I received
Padre Pio and St. Matthew relics and oils from friends. Although
I am not one to go on pilgrimages, I have always respected every
person's religious beliefs and practices.

I believe that spirituality is a personal thing and everyone
should be allowed to practice as he or she chooses. The rosary
was a central part of family life when my generation was growing
up. I put my faith in it, and I visualized Mary the Mother of God

sending a shining light to burn the cancer out of my body.

Paradoxically, I was determined that I would not be ambushed by any God squad or some group of self-appointed apostles who might want to put my cry for pity on their billboard. Neither was I inclined towards investing in shares in the afterlife just yet, because I did not want to go there. I was prepared to pass on the one-way ticket that would take me to that better place on the other side, regardless of how good the facilities there might be. If deals could be done, I wanted a stay of execution on the sentence placed upon me. The better place for me was at home with my family. Towards this outcome, I welcomed everything that came my way, from the lighting of a penny candle to intercessions with whatever greater powers people believed in. I would never dismiss help from any quarter, especially at a time when it seemed that the compass of my future was pointing towards very disturbed waters.

My good friends Richard, Gerry, and Michael were always at hand. Their phone calls and text messages were always welcome, especially when spirits were low or the challenges seemed insurmountable. I was always assured of many texts as I made the short but lonesome walk from the car park into the Cancer Centre. The kindness and generosity of people knew no bounds. Friends and neighbors extended offers from walking the dog to doing our laundry. Fortunately, we did not have to call in the offers. Added to this, a family friend gave me an angel worry box containing three angels to take care of me. They are treasured keepsakes, and I still call upon them when times get tough.

I received mass bouquets, relics, and holy medals, together with get-well cards from many people. I was grateful to everyone who sent me messages of goodwill. Cards and messages of support from the people of my native West Clare particularly tugged at my heart, bringing tears—not of pain but of raw emotion. These people actually cared enough for my family and me in our time of need. I believe that all of this sustained us.

When a family friend and neighbor died in September, 2005, I couldn't get to the funeral because of my hospital commitments. And I was not in a proper emotional state to attend a funeral in my circumstances. I phoned her brother to extend my sympathies. While he appreciated the sentiment of my call, Joe quickly focused on my predicament and gave me a motivationally inspiring pep talk. He told me that I needed to focus on my battle with cancer. He impressed on me that I owed it to my family and myself to dig deep for one almighty effort. Joe assured me that I had what it took to fight now and beat the cancer. He put aside his grief for his sister to lend words of encouragement to me. Joe was always at hand when I needed him.

"Faithless is he that says farewell when the road darkens."
—J.R.R. Tolkien

I was like a grounded ship, incapacitated by my illness, and there was no hiding from that reality. My independence was ripped from me, and I was physically winged. I had to search deep for the resources to keep going on this journey.

I drew inspiration from my late father's favorite poem "Never Say Fail" by Charles Swain. The reward for my endeavors was life itself. My will constantly reassured me when my poor body felt the full impact of the cancer and the medication. I knew that success was somewhere in the Great Out There waiting for me to grasp it. Victory would come in the form of a miraculous recovery and walking away from cancer. It would not come easy. It would require patience, perseverance, and faith in the tsunamis of goodwill together with the prayers people sent heavenward on my behalf.

It would be remiss of me not to acknowledge the role played by my canine Golden Retriever friend Buddy, who was sensitive to my every need and mood, whereupon he would lie beside me or place his chin on my lap as if to say, "Let me share in this journey with you. Together we will conquer 'the emperor of all maladies,'" and so we did.

Excerpted from Kevin Haugh's *An Imperfect Storm*

AM I WEIRD, OR WHAT?

Les Mahler

When I was diagnosed in 2007 and told that this brain cancer "would kill me," I wasn't devastated or hurt. I took a half-hour to cry and then picked myself up and said I would move forward. My attitude about this cancer is that it's not the end-all, not so frightening. "The end of the world" is not here.

And it's not like I haven't been told the same thing over and over again; five oncologists, and all with the same prognosis— this cancer is fatal. Heck, even some of my other doctors have said the same.

Okay, I get it. The cancer is deadly, fatal. But I'm not dead and you can't predict when I'll die. No one can. Besides, and this really helped me, life is fatal. No one will live forever.

It's all about my age. I was fifty-seven when diagnosed, and now I'm sixty-four. Not a child anymore, and I've lived my dream to be a journalist.

Sure, some bad stuff has happened along the way. My four children were kidnapped by their mother, and then I raised them as a single dad for nearly twenty years. I watched my father die of brain cancer at sixty-three years old. I had a son taken away from me when he was a toddler. He wasn't told about me until he was thirteen. He never wants to meet me. That hurts, really hurts.

Yes, doctors did find a new growth. A CT scan this Thursday will tell me what's going on. If it has spread, there's nothing left to do; if it's just one spot, perhaps radiation. Will know more by next week.

I'm betting it's nothing, very manageable. I seldom ever win bets. And if it is manageable, I'll continue with life as best as I can. (The fibromyalgia is worse than the cancer, absolutely lays you down to where you don't want to do anything, just rest.)

But I don't want to waste a day, rest yes, but only for so long, and then it's on to living life as best as possible. There are only so many days in life, and if you lose one, there is no return trip and no making up what you've lost.

So, am I weird or what?

WHAT HELPED MY HEALING?

I guess for me it was attitude, humor. From the very first day of my diagnosis, I would bring in humor to daily radiation treatments. I would ask what type of barbecue sauce I should bring when I was on the table being radiated. I would remind them to get my good side, because "I have many adoring fans." It really was all about not letting the downside win, because then you really would lose out.

Plus, for me, dealing with children with cancer, I realized that I had it good. I had already lived my dreams. I became the journalist that I had dreamt of being. Children were just beginning. I had no reason to complain, no right to complain.

Honestly, if I had to say what helped me most, it was my attitude. I never looked at cancer as anything more than a disease. It wasn't the horror that I had heard about. I was sick, with a disease. Being a journalist, I had a rebellious attitude. If I could take on law enforcement and government officials on a daily basis—and have them fear me because I could expose corruption or wrongdoings—cancer wasn't going to beat me.

Plus, the most important part in this battle was realizing that I am not dead yet. As long as I remembered that, the battle was going my way. If I could put my feet to the floor, and every day, if I woke and saw the morning sun—I was still winning the battle. That was important to me. That's what kept me going.

THE STRONGEST WOMAN IN THE WORLD: A Cancer Allegory

Jack Lagomarsino

She closed her eyes.

She had seen what lay ahead. She hid for a moment in the darkness. Wrapped herself in a deep breath.

She was so calm.

She steadied herself for the road ahead. For the fear and uncertainty. Amidst the confusion, her confidence was radiant. She couldn't sense it, but the world could. The world could feel her poise.

Vulnerable, she lifted her chin towards the heavens, as if to ask for something. She must have asked for strength, and god must have complied; nothing else could have explained the power she possessed. She became an angel as the noonday sun washed over her skin. She could have lifted into the skies at that very moment, but she decided to stay. To use the strength she'd been given.

Despite her confidence, she stood in awe of the task at hand. She had never been faced with such an obstacle. None of us had. She picked up a walking stick and took her first step. A full step closer. The trail was steep and strenuous. Like ribbons, it curled and split into shadows.

Her strides were short but uninterrupted as her will conquered the slopes, rocks and knee-deep puddles. Fallen trees cluttered the path. Constant reminders of those who had lost the battle.

The trail got steeper. Promising toeholds crumbling underfoot. Sharper turns with less visibility. More fallen tree reminders. Her hasty ascent slowed to a crawl as the pressures of the world rained down. She wanted to break. She wanted to cry and roll back down the hill she had worked so hard to conquer.

Instead, she fought to her feet once more. Because she had to. Because her son needed her to. Because she could.

Before trudging on, she took a look at herself and saw something special.

A survivor.

She realized that she had come to the end of the trail. The setting sun once again set an angelic glow to her face and cast away the shadows that had clouded her ascent. Her devotion to life and loyalty to the ones she loved had pulled her through what was undoubtedly the most difficult journey of her life. She breathed deep and fell into the open arms of a world that was praying for her—cheering wildly for the strongest woman in the world.

Written in tribute to his mother Judy Nee,
when Jack was seventeen

WHAT HELPED ME THROUGH

Confidence. From day one, I was confident that my mom would be just fine. I had no reason to be. There were scary moments, close calls, and plenty of setbacks, but I didn't let negative energy or sad, fictional futures work their way into our process. I knew she was going to be okay, and, importantly, that entertaining alternatives was entirely counterproductive. It's so much easier to fight when you're confident you'll win.

CANCER'S GIFTS

"We, too, can learn to be seers—
seers of the blessings, learnings, mercies, and protections
that are ever present on a daily basis."
—Angeles Arrien

YOU ARE NOT YOUR CANCER

Paul Brenner

I am a psychosocial oncologist at the San Diego Cancer Center. I have been living with cancer for fifteen years. One of the most important messages I give to anyone sitting in my office is *You are not your cancer.*

I started as an obstetrician, so I know that a newborn child is not only a miracle, but also love made visible. That essence continues throughout our childhood and into adulthood. Cancer should not and cannot overtake it.

We can never allow cancer to dominate or define who we are.

My patients have taught me so much. I've seen that we are not responsible for creating our illnesses, but we are responsible for responding to them. We can all decrease anxiety, depression, anger, and discomfort, by focusing on spiritual well-being. And that is not a pie-in-the-sky statement. That is a medical fact.

Spiritual well-being can lower your blood pressure and the risk of heart disease, help you adjust to the effects of cancer and its treatment, and increase your ability to enjoy life during cancer treatment. And, as we all know, enjoyment brings more enjoyment.

So please, as best you can, try to resolve the stresses and fears within your life. Observe your thoughts and control those that are negative, fearful, or anxiety-provoking. It's not as hard as it sounds!

Early on, in my struggle with cancer, I realized that a large number of my daily thoughts were unhealthy or focused on the future or the past. With careful attention, I also discovered that my mind could not hold two thoughts at once. I wanted to embrace, not dread, the wonderful world around me. So, rather than let the negative anxieties outweigh the positive ones, I devised skills to remedy the imbalance.

Here is what you do. When a negative or redundant thought fills your mind, simply repeat to yourself a single word. I use the word "delete" over and over again, for about ten seconds. This easy process can cancel negative thoughts for a prolonged period of time. Or, I ask patients to just clap their hands as a distraction. *Negative thoughts, begone!* My favorite negativity stopper, the one that I use myself, is *I am love—that can't be my thought.* I find this phrase cleanses my thought patterns and fills me with calm.

In over fifty years of medical practice, my patients have taught me that fear is the enemy of love. And perhaps most importantly, love is the absence of fear. Think of that baby you once were—love made visible. Don't allow cancer or anything to diminish who you are.

You don't have to let negativity rule your thoughts. You can simply take note, and repeat "delete."

Originally appeared in the *Stand Up to Cancer* newsletter

A MOMENT OF GRACE

Judy Garvey

April 2006. My husband sits with me in my surgeon's office, waiting for her to return. She had just removed a lump from my breast, and was personally conveying it to the lab. My mom died twenty-five years before from breast cancer. I've had several lumps removed from my breasts, all of them benign, but this time is different, and I know it.

My doctor returns, sits down behind her desk, and states the words I've feared all my adult life — "You have cancer." I am thrown upside down, sideways, caught in a tidal wave of grief, terror, and doom. I have no idea which way is up. I can't catch my breath. There's a roaring noise in my ears, blocking out the surgeon's words as she proceeds to tell us the cellular breakdown of my particular cancer.

For ten long minutes, I am tossed, turned, thrown about, struggling to find a way out of my panic, to a place where I can breathe. But I'm lost . . . helpless . . . hopeless. Living the nightmare I dreaded for twenty-five long years.

Then, a single sentence forms in my mind, *Thank God, I found it now.*

And with this simple thought of gratitude, calm washes

through my body, from head to toe, in an almost physical wave. I return to myself, as if awakening from a horrible dream. My body still sits in the chair in my doctor's office and my feet solidly touch the floor. But now I am back—determined and clear. I know that this feeling of peace, this moment of clarity, is a part of my deepest being now and always. In my darkest moments, I'll be able to feel gratitude—for early detection, for this day, and for these moments of grace.

And so, that day in my doctor's office, I made the commitment to fight for my health and my life. Taking a deep breath, I asked, "What do we do next?"

WHAT WORKED FOR ME

Living my life day to day (not wanting to waste any good days worrying about the potentially scary future)

My awesome husband Larry, my slightly crazy dog Sadie, and our semi-feral cat Shyster

Visualizations of driving my racecar (and winning)

Multi-colored bandanas (I bought a wig, but never wore it)

Meditation for Dummies CD

Watermelon

The Serenity Prayer on a bookmark

Listening to books on tape

Feeling confident about doing things my way and listening to my instincts

Setting firm limits about listening to other people's fears and sometimes-clueless advice

Breathing/grounding techniques (feeling my feet on the floor, breathing in and out slowly, centering myself in my core)

Creating a strong team feeling with my surgeon and oncologist

Seeing the humor in things and trying to laugh as often as possible

BEATING THE ODDS

Neil A. Fiore

Thirty-five years ago, I was given a 10 percent chance of living one more year.

When my doctor told me that I had cancer that had spread to my left lung, and that he had already scheduled surgery to remove my right testicle the following morning, I heard myself say, "No, doctor, surgery is not scheduled for tomorrow morning." I told him I wanted a second and third opinion, and that I needed to speak with my family. I was just thirty-two years old.

The doctor responded, "Some people are afraid of dying, including me."

Once again, I heard myself respond—as if I were watching and listening from a distance—"Doctor, I'm not afraid of dying, but I am afraid of what your fear of cancer will do to me."

I had already confronted my fear of death ten years earlier during paratrooper training and in Vietnam with the 101st Airborne Division. But that didn't lessen the shock of hearing a "terminal" cancer diagnosis. My mind raced with thoughts of how to cope with the odds I had been given. I could accept that having metastasized cancer could lead to death in one year, but I decided right there in that doctor's office that it was going to be one hell of a year and one terrific fight.

If I had only one year to live, I was determined to not live it in fear and on his schedule. I would not be following the orders of a doctor who had scheduled surgery without consulting me, the patient. I wanted to participate in the treatment decisions that were going to affect my life.

I asked the doctor what research he based his decision on. He was gracious enough to tell me, and I took down the names of the medical journals he cited and went directly to the hospital's medical library.

After about four hours of research in the medical library, I came to the conclusion that there was no miracle cure for my type of cancer. The first treatment stage for my cancer was exploratory surgery to be followed by the removal of lymph nodes in an eight-hour operation. Preliminary tests found, however, that the cancer was not "spreading" through my lymph nodes. Now I was prepared to argue with the chief surgeon that I no longer needed the dreaded eight-hour surgery to remove most of my lymph nodes. In fact, new x rays showed a second spot in my left lung indicating that any "spreading" was clearly through my blood stream. I was ready to reason with the surgeon that cancer doesn't just spread through the lymph nodes and to the lungs as if the body is passive. The body's immune system actively captures and holds cancer cells in the lymph nodes and the lungs filter the blood of debris.

But he had a surprise for me. He told me that he could remove the bottom lobe of my left lung. I insisted that since we had evidence of spreading through the bloodstream, I needed chemotherapy that goes into my blood stream. If he removed my lung, that wouldn't stop the spread of cancer through the rest of my blood stream, but would only leave me with half of my filtering system. He said, "You have a point there." With that remark, I pounded my fist on his desk and said, "I want chemotherapy today!"

Fortunately, the experimental chemotherapy protocol I started saved my lung and my life. It was the first chemotherapy that worked on stopping testicular cancers, and 80 percent of us on that protocol survived. Since then, newer chemotherapies have raised the survival rate to 90 percent.

I admit that I was an unusually active patient, but remember, I was fighting for my life against really overwhelming odds. It amazed my doctors that I would actually argue to get chemotherapy when most patients resisted taking these powerful drugs. But I believe that precisely because I had to fight to get the chemotherapy, I was free of side effects for the first two months. My body was able to lower its stress hormones and to work with the chemotherapy, because I was fully choosing to consider the chemotherapy as a powerful ally.

When my hair eventually began to fall out, I told myself that my medicine was working to kill rapidly dividing cells and the loss of hair was evidence of that, given that hair cells are some of the fastest growing cells.

Yes, my methods were somewhat unusual, but I was on a mission to speak up for those patients who are less assertive than I am. My doctors and I became a team, and they asked me to make a video to show other patients how to cope with chemotherapy and its side effects. When that seemed to help, they asked me to speak to the rest of the doctors at Grand Rounds.

I believe I survived the odds because of expert surgery and chemotherapy and because I argued with my doctors. All three contributed to saving my life. Had I been passive, I would have died that first year.

Since then, I counsel people diagnosed with cancer to ask questions, gather whatever information they need to make informed decisions, and then fully choose their treatment. This relaxes your body during treatment, lowers the stress hormones, can lessen side effects, and allows your body to recover more quickly.

I wish you well in confronting your own odds with the knowledge that even if given only a 10 percent chance, as I was given, when you're in that 10 percent, you're 100 percent alive.

WHAT SUPPORTED MY HEALING

I was supported by my own stubbornness, and my refusal to passively accept the doctor's limited view of the human body's ability to fight cancer cells along with surgery and chemotherapy.

My training in self-hypnosis helped me enormously to identify the words of "negative hypnosis" that came from others and myself, and to reach deep levels of relaxation for rapid recuperation.

Friends and therapy helped me to express my feelings and to keep me from feeling alone.

Nutrition was a neglected aspect of the medical treatment, so I consulted with someone to help the healthy part of me stay strong enough to clear very strong chemotherapeutic agents, and to help mop up any remaining cancer cells.

Writing for future cancer patients and speaking up for others who were not as assertive as I was gave me a mission. It encouraged me to speak up even more against practices that I felt harmed the ability of patients to maintain reasonable hope.

WHEN THE PERFORMANCE STOPS
Shariann Tom

I'm tired. I need a break. I can't seem to keep up this pace, this face. I'm not being real to everyone. I'm pretending that I'm unaffected by what is happening. "I've got it handled," is the persona I try to portray, hoping that this will help them look at me less pathetically. Their brows furrow and their eyes seem to plead with me. "How are you doing?" they ask. I know they think they want to know, but I don't think they can handle the truth. I don't think I could bear their pity-look or pity-voice if I told them the truth.

"I feel like crap," I'd say, if I could. "I'm scared that my future is limited, and I'm sad that I have to go through this treatment that makes me feel like sh-t." Would they be able to stand behind me and rally? Or would they say that dreaded phrase, "It will all be okay." And, that isn't even the deep dark truth. The truth is that I feel so alone, because I can't be with where I am, not even with myself. So, the mask of "I'm fine" is for them as well as me.

I go on pretending to them and to myself. I pretend that everything is progressing well. I pretend that I have it all together and do not want to curl up into a ball and sleep for a million hours. I pretend that this is a detour of my life, but really it feels

176

like I got kicked off the path and ejected to the path of doom and gloom. A penance for a life of too many Cheetos and hours of useless TV? Did I take on too much stress, more than my body could handle, and it was now rebelling? Was I wasting my life away and this was its way of getting my attention?

Whatever brought the cancer here doesn't matter. I'm awake. Awake with impatience and annoyance. I want this done, complete. I want to have energy again. I want to not be tired. With a sigh, I realize that this is not the way to get past the tiredness. Beating myself up just takes more energy; energy that I don't have. I surrender into the weariness of it all and release holding my body up and sink into the chair that is under me. I feel the sadness coursing through me, as if tracking through my veins. I let the tears come, as I hold my head in my hands. The tears feel good, like rain that washes the pavement clean. This is real. This feels better.

I have been a performer, all my life: performing for the approval of my parents, inclusion of my siblings, and belonging with my friends. I didn't feel that I would be truly loved, being myself. So I was the good daughter, the I'll-follow-you-anywhere sister, and the do-what-everyone-else-is-doing girlfriend. I wasn't even sure who the real me was, I had performed for so long. Cancer stopped this.

Here is the gift, the miracle I received. I didn't have any energy for the performance and pretense, anymore. The physical devastation stripped me raw, and all I could do was be who was right here—the real essence of me. There was no time for playing it safe or nice or for someone else. And, in this raw place of surrender, I discovered me. I discovered the parts that were naturally me without effort, and my genuine opinions, likes and dislikes. I discovered what I was made of—my natural strengths and my personal values. I discovered that I loved me, and my real healing began.

HOW I MADE IT THROUGH THE WORRIES

1. *My team signed up on my schedule, and I had someone different (with some repeats) of friends and family who would join me for my appointments for doctor visits, scans, tests, etc. Having someone there made the event more entertaining, because I got to visit with someone rather than sit there alone. My companion also helped either distract me or discuss with me whatever was happening in the moment, so I didn't have to carry it or push it down. These human allies really were human angels.*

2. *Having a compelling vision that excited me. We all don't know when we will leave this earth and that shouldn't stop us from allowing ourselves to dream and envision a future vision that excites and calls us. Through my various cancer journeys, I had different visions, but they were bigger than the cancer and bigger than getting through the cancer. One was seeing myself as the mommy I always wanted to be for my children and to experience their big moments. That came from being there in their small moments: graduations, performances, and all the times when they reached beyond who they thought they were. We were surprised and delighted. Allowing myself to see these future moments in my mind's eye in Technicolor helped me reach for life beyond cancer.*

3. *I've learned that loving myself with compassion, patience, and gentleness (the way that I love my children) means giving myself what is needed and not looking for someone or something outside of me to do it. Learning how to nourish and nurture myself when anxiety and panic showed up was one of the greatest gifts that I could give myself. The most healing thing I learned to do was the "knowing" that I would not abandon myself, and that I would always be there for me, always focusing on what was best for me. I am kinder to myself and to the world because of this.*

I hope these help.

MY CANCER AND MY SON

Laurie Hessen Pomeranz

On the day before my mastectomy, I went to visit my Dad. I wanted to give him a hug, to reassure him I was okay, and to see in his face that he believed I'd be okay.

When we said good-bye, the anguish in his eyes was unmistakable. I said, "Dad, I'm going to be fine. I'm not scared. I'm in good hands. Please, don't be scared." He gazed at me with his trademark gentleness, and said, "Sweetheart, if someone accidentally elbowed you, I'd be upset . . . and this is much bigger than that."

In that moment, I realized in a whole new, visceral way how much we suffer at the thought of our child suffering.

When I learned that I had breast cancer, I was dreading the pain and fear it would cause my boy, Jack. He already knew about cancer because my mother died of the disease fourteen years before he was born. I knew that in his mind, he would make the association with his Grandma Bea, and imagine his mama might die, too.

My husband, Jeff, and I did not disclose the news of my diagnosis for a week or so, until we knew what the action plan would be. Then, it was time to tell our son. On a sunny Sunday afternoon, we sat Jack down and I got started. I told him I'd seen and felt a funny bump in my breast, so I went to the doctor and he took a little piece out of it, and we found out it was cancer. I would have surgery and then some very strong medicine that would make the cancer go away.

Jack stared into the distance and said, "Whoa. You have cancer?" Long pause. "Whoa . . . "

We explained the cancer I had was very different than the cancer his Grandma Bea had in her kidney. I was lucky, because I could feel the bump and get it taken out. Grandma's cancer wasn't one you could see or feel, so no one knew until it was too late.

I looked into Jack's thoughtful blue eyes, eyes far-away and churning with new information, and I asked, "How are you feeling right now?" He stared back at me, and said, "I kind of just feel like, whoa . . . " A long, heavy pause followed, and then, "Can we go outside and play catch now?" With a little laugh of surprise and relief, I said, "That sounds like a great idea, buddy." I was struck by my child's ability to know how much he could tolerate for the moment. After a week of diagnostic work-ups—a mammogram, CT scan, ultrasound, PET scan, MRI, and several grueling biopsies—I was bruised and scared, and playing catch was exactly what I needed to keep me feeling like life would go on. Jack was approaching and retreating from the intensity in just the way he needed, and it was a revelation to me.

Ultimately, I completed eight months of treatment that included a mastectomy, four months of chemotherapy, and six weeks of radiation. The rigors of cancer treatment impacted my mothering and my ability to be available to Jack in all the ways I normally am. Because he's my only child, he has received the entirety of my maternal attention. But during the exhausting months of treatment, I needed to allocate significantly more time and attention to my own needs.

I could not chaperone field trips, or be room mom at school, or play catch in the backyard, or shoot hoops at the park. We had to find new, more calm, less strenuous ways to be together. There were incisions, drains, bone pains, steroids that kept me up all night, anti-nausea meds that made me sleep all day, and radiation burns. There was no roughhousing, no getting scrappy. Jack had to be careful around me. Mama was much more delicate than usual. Before he'd lie down next to me and rest his head against my chest, he'd ask, "Can I put my head right here?"

Having cancer made me want to hold fast to my husband and son. Embracing my boy was even more poignant and crucial than ever. I felt physically, emotionally, and mentally calmer when he was close, and I could hold his warm, skinny body against mine. My husband described an emotion that often swept over him, to want to hold our son, and me, tighter than ever. Family snuggles became a biological imperative.

An upside of my new fragility was that we did a lot of quiet cuddling in bed and on the pullout couch, where we often set up camp for dinner. Cancer made me eat only anti-processed food and anti-empty carbs, so hot dogs and mac n' cheese were off the table. I don't recommend getting cancer for this, but an amazing by-product of my weakened state was that people cooked for us—often and fabulously. We were treated to healthy, beautiful vegetarian dinners made by an incredible, far-reaching circle of friends: our village in the big city. And, we came to deeply appreciate a new facet of Jack's adaptable personality, as he dove into plates of Chinese five-spice tofu and Mexican quinoa salad.

For the four days after each chemo treatment, I was bedridden with bone pain. Jeff nicknamed me "Shuffley" for the way I would totter across the bedroom floor, to the kitchen, and then back to bed. It was very difficult to have Jack in the house during those dark days. It felt like my bones were in labor. I required a lot of silence, sleep, and pain medication to get through it.

We needed to ask for a lot of help with Jack. He went for sleepovers and play dates far more often than usual, and with a wider range of friends and family than ever before. I came to know and respect Jack's sense of adventure in a whole new way, as I watched him pack up his little SpongeBob wheelie bag and head out with wide eyes and enthusiasm to a medley of different homes. He always came back with funny stories to tell about his friends' little brothers and sisters and their antics, especially at the dinner table.

Letting Jack go, trusting that he could feel safe, happy, and secure with so many caring people was probably as valuable a learning experience for us as it was for him. We had to let him go, and be ready to receive him—to give him a sense of home and stability when he returned. It was good preparation for the rest of our lives as parents.

At the one-year anniversary of my diagnosis, my cancerversary, I asked Jack what he thought had been different about the previous year, when I was sick. He said, "You couldn't play sports with me . . . but now you're better!" I am indeed. It feels like a miracle.

Makes me want to go outside and play catch.

Originally appeared in *The Mother Company*, 2011, and in
*The Day My Nipple Fell Off and Other Stories of Survival,
Solidarity, and Sass: a BAYS Anthology*, 2013

WHAT HELPED ME THROUGH THE ANGST

During the darkest, most grueling days of treatment, I relied on a number of things to help me keep going. First and foremost, I learned to say "yes" to any and all offers of tangible, practical, and emotional support! Letting friends and neighbors cook for me and my family, sit by my side at chemo, lie in my bed with me while I recovered, drive my son places and take him for play dates and sleepovers . . . all were invaluable.

Finding and deeply connecting with the women of the Bay Area Young Survivors, a local support group, gave me a sisterhood who knew, intimately, what I was feeling and thinking about. I never felt alone.

Lastly, keeping joy in my life was crucial to surviving the rigors of cancer. I continued to sing and dance with my band throughout treatment, slapping on different colored wigs for every gig. Just feeling the joy and vitality in my body during concerts helped me to remember that I was still in there, despite how differently I looked and felt much of the time. As a family, we enjoyed the delicious, nearly daily distraction of the San Francisco Giants' march to the World Series, which served the powerful function of letting us lose ourselves and have fun together, all the while lying down on the couch.

OPPORTUNITY KNOCKS
Judith Cohen

I was diagnosed with both ovarian and endometrial cancers in October of 1998. It's hard to believe that sixteen years have passed since that fateful day. Thankfully, I've been cancer free since my treatment. In order to augment my own healing, I decided early on to use my skills as a clinical social worker and transformation coach to support other cancer patients—to help them deal not only with their diagnoses but also to work through the many strong emotions that arise in the face of cancer. I also spent many hours involved in advocacy and community education, and coached over a hundred cancer patients in the first years after my own diagnosis. I not only survived, but I have thrived due to a rigorous treatment protocol, the support of family, friends, colleagues, and even complete strangers.

As a complete stranger, may I tell you what I learned?

For a good seven years, my life was totally focused on cancer and the effects of my year-long treatment. I remember the wrenching stomach pain in 1998 that sent me to my doctor. And the two-week wait between my sonogram and my surgery, when I had to seriously consider that I might be ill. Then, ten days after exploratory surgery, my surgeon said, "I'm sorry to have to tell you—" and I stopped listening. Fortunately, a good friend who had accompanied me to the doctor's appointment heard the end of the sentence, "—that I found cancer in both your ovary and uterus."

Shocked, I remember looking at my watch, thinking I'd die in a few minutes. Who could live with a dual diagnosis like that?

Luckily, my surgeon had optimistic odds for my survival. "80/20," he said. "I'm going for a complete cure!"

I told my friends and family, "I am going into the cancer monastery for a year. When I come out, I'll be healed in mind, body, and spirit." It was an excellent metaphor. Like monks who enter monasteries to meditate and study, I shaved my head and shed my everyday behaviors to pay full attention to my treatment. Yes, of course, I grieved, but in time I found a way to turn that grief into a gift that helped me take stock of my life and make decisions about what mattered most. I created my own healing narrative during this cancer sabbatical. I contemplated who I was and who I wanted to be. What rose to the top? Service to others and compassionate love for myself.

No matter how awful I felt as my treatment wore on, and it was severe, I turned the experience into a quest to help other cancer patients. As a participant/observer, I became rigorously curious about my pain, and what alleviated it, so I could share those tips with others. And I focused my coaching business on working with newly diagnosed patients, applying what I called "chemo coaching." I told clients that their quest was to face treatments so that they could understand their own strengths and develop powerful coping mechanisms. The terrible scare of cancer makes us open to change. As a total believer in the mind/

body connection, I helped so many people change their stories of tragedy into stories of possibility, directed by their own core purposes and desires.

Although I never want to have to deal with cancer again, ironically it was the perfect answer to so many of my prayers. I learned that I was resilient, could face death and grief with equanimity and grace, and most importantly that the choices I made in life directly determined how happy or unhappy I would be. I used to joke with my therapist that, even though she was the best therapist in the world, cancer had her beat. It was far more effective because it had no interest in my rationalizations and distortions. It had only one commitment and that was to annihilate me in the service of its own life.

I doubt that I am alone in having this experience. I do think that it is a perk of cancer that shouldn't be overlooked. My mantra before cancer was, "There's no point in experiencing a tragedy if you can't make it work for you!" My mantra after cancer shifted to, "There's no point in having cancer if you can't use your experience to help others."

When opportunity knocks, make it work for you.

WHAT HELPED ME THROUGH THE ANGST AND ANGUISH

The most important things were not things but people. Allow people to help you. I was single when I was diagnosed, but between my friends, family, colleagues, medical team, and strangers, I grew a community around me. Most people are healing and want to help. And if you don't know anyone, join a sup-

port group, either through your treatment facility or a freestanding support service such as The Wellness Community (now called Cancer Support Community in some cities). Your oncology social worker should be able to provide you with resources. Talk to other patients while you're getting your chemo. See what they're doing for support as well.

Humor. Although comedians do talk about their success as "I killed . . ." and their failure at getting laughs as "I died . . ." humor saved my life. Being able to see the humor in the often absurd situations that cancer offers you will definitely help your healing. One great thing about cancer was that it got me to do standup comedy. I was dying anyway, so I had nothing to lose! I performed at Grand Rounds for the nurses and at an American Cancer Society fundraiser.

Therapy or coaching can provide much solace and healing. My therapist was willing to laugh at me during some particularly dark times. She lightened my mood and reminded me to not take myself so seriously, even if I were dying. She also cried with me and helped me hold my grief, not only for my own loss of my previous life but for the deaths of the many people I had come to know and love in the community.

Web Resources—
Steve Dunn's Cancer Guide (www.cancerguide.org). Unfortunately, Steve died from complications of bacterial meningitis in 2005, but he was cancer free for fifteen years after his diagnosis of stage IV (terminal) kidney cancer. He wrote an incredibly detailed and helpful guide for people just getting diagnosed with any form of cancer. He has articles on what questions to ask, the meaning of

statistics, and other issues of concern to newly diagnosed people. This site is his legacy.

I worked for almost a year at the National Cancer Institute's Cancer Information Service (www.cancer.gov). You can call them Monday to Friday from 8 A.M. to 8 P.M. (ET) and ask any question you want. The service is available in English and Spanish. You can download information on all sorts of cancer treatments, nutrition, symptoms, etc. at their site. Your tax dollars are paying for this information, so make use of this free service for cancer patients and their families.

I found an incredible amount of support at the Association of Cancer Online Resources (www.acor.org). This is a group of Listservs divided by diagnosis for patients, caregivers, friends, etc. It is open 24/7 and you can not only get answers to all sorts of questions—like, "How do I tell my clients I have cancer?" and other questions not usually talked about in cancer guides—but you can also make good friends. I actually ended up meeting two of the women I corresponded with in person, and I stayed in connection for many years after my treatment ended.

Caring Bridge (www.caringbridge.org) is another place to get support. You can write about how you're doing, and your friends and family can get updates and write in to you offering support, jokes, etc. If you're too sick to write, you can also have someone else give updates and share the information that you want shared. Lotsa Helping Hands (www.lotsahelpinghands.com) is an organizing site for caregivers. Assign one person to oversee the tasks that need to be done each week (food, drive to chemo, cleaning, etc.), and then let her or him post the tasks that are open and allow people to sign up and help you. You don't have to think about anything, and your friends can be useful and actually help you out in an orderly way.

RED BADGE OF COURAGE

Kelly Gallaher Greene

In 1992, my whole world came screeching to a halt, and I came face to face with my mortality. A laryngoscopy revealed cancerous tumors in my throat. My doctor said that radiation would give me an 85 percent chance of total recovery. I was so shocked; I couldn't even ask an intelligent question. Like, "Are you sure you have the right patient?"

My husband and I cried together. My family was stunned silent. I realized, driving to work the next day, how depressed I had been for a long time. I felt trapped in an unhappy marriage. I worried about thinly stretched finances. And facing an empty nest, as my daughter would be leaving for college. *How will we pay for that? How will I survive her absence?* But suddenly, my almost unbearable existence looked—well, all right. In fact, it seemed just fine, thank you very much. *I'll take it!* I wanted to be alive. I was nearly ecstatic to be driving on this fabulous crowded freeway heading to my wonderful job.

During the nine weeks of radiation treatment, as I cycled in and out of episodes of sickening panic, two other powerful insights came. I decided I had to come face to face with my fear. It was certainly time. I felt I couldn't confront it on my own, so

I asked my husband to simply hold me while I stared into the eyes of death.

We sat on the couch together as I closed my eyes and let total darkness envelop me. My consciousness began dissolving into a black void. Sobs shook my body. I stayed with this terrible fear until the tears finally subsided. I felt completely exhausted. Empty. Then an odd sense of calm, almost peace, came over me. I saw clearly that the images I had conjured were pure fantasy. All imagination. Just something I made up. When I faced what I feared most—"nothingness"—it vanished. Just like the monster in my childhood nightmares, the paralyzing fear was gone.

The second insight came so unexpectedly! Through a psychic, someone I would never ordinarily have called. When a friend suggested I consult her psychic healer in Florida, the idea seemed like a lifeline. I dialed the phone. This brusque stranger was so matter-of-fact. When she heard I was calling about a cancer diagnosis, she softened a little. She said, "You're going to be okay." And that this was a karmic lesson I had chosen prior to my birth. Then she told me, "Go through the radiation treatments and surrender to them completely. Get out of the way of the healing. Surround yourself with positive things and people. Pray and meditate every day." And she assured me the cancer would not spread.

This ten-minute phone call flipped me out of victimhood. I didn't question it or doubt what the psychic had said. It felt miraculous. It was all about having faith and never letting it waver.

And so I used these three enlivening insights to steer me through the nine hard weeks. Halfway through my radiation sessions, the doctor upgraded my prognosis to a 95 percent chance of total recovery. I was cautiously elated. During the last few weeks, I could actually feel the radiation entering my throat, even though they assured me I shouldn't be able to. As the tissue broke down, a rectangular patch that looked like a sunburn began forming on my neck, getting darker and darker. It was tender, like a burn. I thought of it as my badge of healing and courage.

Looking back now, twenty years later, I know this cancer battle taught me so much about my body and myself. Cancer changed my whole point of view. The dull mundanity of everyday reality was ripped away like a curtain on a stage, and I saw how precarious and precious life really is. I found courage. I am so grateful. Courage and gratitude have dynamic power.

Magic happens when I remember to give thanks for all of the miracles in my life.

METHODS I USED TO STAY CALM AND PEACEFUL

When I was diagnosed with throat cancer, I went into a tailspin. All of my fears about death and dying flew into my face, and I felt totally helpless and terrified. Through an amazing shift in attitude, I was able to surrender to the process and call upon my friends and loved ones to hold my hand.

I eliminated any and all negativity, both in my own mind and surrounding me. I refused to allow the fear to take over. I meditated and took care of my body with healthy food and exercise. I became aware that my life was a gift, and I practiced gratitude almost like a religion. It was a little prayer I would say in the morning or evening, finding five things I was grateful for every day.

I was gentle with myself and decided not to feel sorry for myself, soon after my fear had subsided.

AFTERWORD – I BOUGHT A PEACOCK
Paige Davis

For the last several months, I have been in serious purging mode. I would imagine this is a common step for people once they emerge from the cancer cocoon and step into this thing called "the new normal." As I begin to gain more energy and vitality every day, I better appreciate the burden and hardship that my body went through as it struggled to heal during my year with cancer. I also realize the mental and energetic toll that my psyche went through. On the positive, I felt real transformation and energetic release. On the negative, I felt like all that energy that had been released was now stuck in my home.

So I tapped into my toolbox of transformation, and I took action to transform my once cancer-centric home into a new space that would set the stage for my best chance of stepping into my new normal.

I tapped into my good ol' days of being a feng shui consultant and got to work. It took several weeks of purging, reorganizing, a little bit of redecorating, and some serious sage burning, but I infused my home inside and out with more vitality (literally bringing in more fire element of reds and oranges), intention, clarity, and freeing up more space—lots and lots of space.

The thing with empty space is, it can be uncomfortable. And I found myself wanting to fill it ASAP, perusing online shopping websites looking for the perfect accessories to "fill it up." But if there was anything I learned through my year with cancer it is that if I can sit in the discomfort and invite a little surrender, the right thing, person, or circumstance will show up exactly when I need it.

Sure enough, a few weeks later, I was running some errands and stumbled upon this completely random store. It was next door to the pet store where I go all the time for my dog, but I never saw it. I was walking by, and I noticed this metal peacock. It was big, heavy, bright, and clunky. Not at all my aesthetic, but it literally stopped me in my tracks, and I thought to myself, I have to have that. I tried to disregard it, because it really was pretty tacky. So I proceeded with my errands, but I couldn't get that peacock out of my head. Sure enough—I went back to the store, and I bought the peacock having no real idea where it would go. Technically, it was described as yard art (I don't even really have a yard), but I recognized this deeper feeling of validation in my soul that I have learned to listen to and follow.

I've always been one for looking at the deeper meaning of things and objects, so of course, the first thing I did, before I bought the peacock, was Google its meaning. Evidently, in many ancient traditions, the peacock was thought to have the power of resurrection, symbolizing renewal and immortality. It is also described as being a symbol of integrity and beauty if we endeavor to express and show our true colors. Hmm—that seemed pretty spot on. It really was the ideal embodiment of where I was emotionally, physically, and spiritually. So now,

196

every time I pull up to my home or my dog pees on that peacock, I am reminded to let my true colors shine through and be kind to myself as I continue to reinvent my reality.

Needless to say, like most symbols, once we become aware, I began to see the peacock in everything. It was in a decorative pillow I bought months earlier. It was in clothing that I had never even noticed. It was featured in random art I began to take notice of. There were TV specials—all about peacocks!

Instead of seeing these things as random, I'm choosing to embrace these little signs, however silly or insignificant they may seem, as little "atta girls" from the universe, reminding me that I'm never really alone. And that circumstances, people, and random objects show up to remind us what we need to know in the moment.

And so as I continue to embrace that it's not about figuring out or doing anything specific to step into my new normal, but rather it is about embracing that I'm actually in it—I'm realizing I don't need the cancer or the treatments or the surgeries to take pause, appreciate, nurture, and love. It's not about doing but rather being these things—through and through. After all, we are human beings, not human doings. Sometimes it just takes something like a tacky peacock to serve as the reminder.

Originally appeared in *The Huffington Post*, 2014

CONTRIBUTORS

These essays are all love letters offering you our hands and hearts. They will walk with you along your journey, as long and as hard as it may be. The authors are all caring supporters who send their best.

Steven Baum is a son, husband, and father. He is inspired by his mother, Nancy Novack, a stage IV cancer survivor, who is living proof that spirit and strength conquer all. He lives in Manhattan Beach, California, with his amazing and beautiful wife, Carrie, and their two Jedi knights, Sebastian and Alexandra.

Dr. Paul Brenner, a renowned physician and psychosocial oncologist, began his career as a gynecologist. During a sabbatical, Paul serendipitously began to counsel patients with life-threatening illnesses. As a result, he stopped practicing medicine in traditional ways and saw one person a day with a chronic or terminal illness.

Fascinated by how emotions integrate the mind and body, Paul obtained a doctorate in counseling psychology, and studied healing in South America, Taiwan, and China. For the past fifty years, he has been in search of "what makes an individual chronically ill or well." His book *Buddha in the Waiting Room* (New Age Books, 2003) tells of this quest to redefine health as a living process. He has appeared on public television and moderated the award-winning KPBS series *Healing Through Communication.*

Aisling Carroll was born and raised in San Francisco. A former Washington, D.C., reporter, she has worked in politics and marketing. At the age of thirty-two and living in Dublin, Ireland, she was diagnosed with ovarian cancer. Luckily, the chemo knocked out the cancer, and she is now clawing her way back to the well world—one doctor, drug, and hot roller at a time. She occasionally types for *The Huffington Post.*

A certified coach and social worker, *Judith Cohen* trains professional coaches and entrepreneurs around the world when fear, self-doubt, and shame sabotage their ability to grow their businesses and create fulfilling relationships. As a senior faculty member of the Coaches Training Institute, Judith has trained over a thousand coaches in her twenty-year career. Writing for *I Am with You* is important to her, because she believes that cancer (no matter the outcome) can help totally change a person's beliefs about what is possible in life, for the better. She says, "Cancer is a disease, and it is also a powerful tool for healing and success, if you allow it to be."
The Opportunity Game (www.theopportunitygame.com)

Paige Davis received a B.A. in Journalism and Environmental Science from the University of Indiana. She is an entrepreneur and co-founded the sustainable lifestyle product company BlueAvocado, which provides thoughtful designs that reduce waste and inspire small steps so that we can all live a greener, simpler life. BlueAvocado is a certified B Corp, with national distribution.

Paige is also a certified meditation teacher with the McLean Meditation Institute and is passionate about inspiring change from a personal place of awareness. She recently created Soul Sparks as a destination to inspire and empower anyone looking to create a meaningful and accessible approach to living a more mindful life through meditation and mindfulness programs.

Paige Davis (www.paigedavis.com)
The Sunshine Chronicles (thesunshinechronicles.blogspot.com)
Souls Sparks (www.SoulSparks.com)

Daphne D. Evans is the founder and CEO of Heaven's Door Cancer Foundation. She is also a CFO startup advisor to various companies in the Bay Area and around the country. She has been a manager and controller consultant to law firms and e-commerce corporations for nearly twenty years. She is a multi-cancer survivor and has been in remission since 2010. As a fundraiser, public speaker, and philanthropist, Daphne has served on the Board of Directors of the Springfield Leukemia & Lymphoma Society.

Daphne's parents, Reverend Donald and Mrs. Ida Evans, have been her inspiration, teaching her that to help others was a ministry that was not passé. Daphne started volunteering to care for those in need at an early age. She helped deliver clothing over bombed-out roads in Nicaragua after the Sandinista regime fell. She hosted clothing drives in San Francisco during the tsunami and found pilots to fly the supplies to the victims there. Daphne also found jobs for young professionals stranded by Katrina and paid out of pocket to fly them to their new job locations. She now hosts fashion shows for fundraising, pairing ladies battling cancer with professional models to walk the runway together. Daphne could never have had the courage or the tenacity to do any of this without her parents showing her that "it is more

blessed to give than to receive."
Heavens Door Cancer Foundation (www.heavensdooropen.com)

Neil B. Feldman is an electrical engineer. He founded two companies that took technical innovation in film production to new heights. He enjoys pioneering innovations in his field, and helped develop the first completely realistic and practical process for converting flat two-dimensional films or videos into stereographic 3D. While studying at Case Western, Neil helped establish the public radio station WCPN. Since that time, he has worked at Motorola in Florida and Third Coast Video in Austin. Neil is one of the few individuals in America to win a case under the FCC's Fairness Doctrine.

Neil has served the Society of Motion Picture and Television Engineers in a variety of positions, including Governor for the Southern Region, and later as Financial Vice President. He is also an active amateur radio operator and a private pilot.

Cindy Finch, MSW, LICSW, is a professional cancer survivor and columnist for Reimagine.me. She has worked at the Mayo Clinic and specializes in supporting patients and families journeying through terminal or traumatic illnesses. She knows a thing or three about this as a cancer survivor and former heart/lung patient. When not with her three children, she enjoys public speaking and developing educational symposiums on a variety of health and survival topics.

Neil A. Fiore—I am a psychologist and a thirty-five-year survivor of a "terminal cancer" diagnosis. I feel a connection to all cancer patients and survivors, and want to offer examples of how they might cope to possibly improve the quality of their care and the chances of their survival. I also want to speak to physicians and nurses about supporting the active participation of their patients, and the holistic treatment of the patient—mind, body, spirit, and emotions. The treatment of cancer must be more than just the elimination of the cancer; it is a process that has to support the healthy aspects of the patient in a joint fight against this deadly disease.

My book, *Coping with the Emotional Impact of Cancer* (Bay Tree Publishing, 2009), tells my story in the introduction, and then takes the family through the various stages and challenges. *Neil Fiore (www.neilfiore.com)*

Dr. Jerome Freedman is an author, mindfulness meditation teacher, and a cancer survivor since 1997. He is a long-time practitioner in the tradition of Zen Master Thich Nhat Hanh in which he is an ordained member of the Order of Interbeing. Jerome served on the Board of Directors of the Marin AIDS Project and the Advisory Council of the Institute for Health and Healing between 2007 and 2010. He holds a Ph.D. in computer science, along with two master's degrees in physics and a bachelor of chemical engineering. His latest book, *Stop Cancer in Its Tracks: How to Embrace Mindfulness in Healing*, was published by CreateSpace in 2014.

Jerome's contribution to *I Am with You* was motivated by leading the practice group at the Pine Street Clinic and seventeen years of guiding cancer patients using the Seven Principles of Mindfulness in Healing. This is also the title of his upcoming book. Having just gone through another eight months of cancer treatments and now being cancer free, Dr. Freedman is learning more about how meditation furthers one's chances of getting through the difficult times with equanimity. Through his publications and his blog, Meditation Practices, he hopes to reach many people who don't know where to turn for guidance in their treatment.

Meditation Practices for Healing and Well-being
www.mountainsangha.org

Judy Garvey—When I was diagnosed with cancer, I was determined to speak up and be an advocate for my health and my life. My diagnosis has changed me in so many positive ways—I'm happier, more mindful of my moment-to-moment existence, and trying my best not to be afraid of the unknown future. I love being connected with enthusiastic people and projects that exude positive energy, so I knew immediately I wanted to be a part of this book project.

Judy Garvey (www.judygarvey.weebly.com)

When *Mark Garza's* father was diagnosed with Stage IV cancer, Mark felt the impact of a diagnosis firsthand. Seeking support, Mark was shocked at the cost of therapy and realized there was a lack of care for thousands of people who were going through similar experiences. He teamed up with The LIVESTRONG Foundation to fill the void for a streamlined process that would provide families in need with financial assistance to access long-term psychological help. Their first fundraiser in 2010, Dam That Cancer, raised over $32,000 for the cause. Mark then founded The Flatwater Foundation, a nonprofit dedicated to providing emotional support to Austin families impacted by cancer. The twelve-plus years of global advertising and event marketing Mark did prior to founding The Flatwater Foundation

serve him well in this creative, inspiring work.
The Flatwater Foundation (www.flatwaterfoundation.org)

My name is *Sue Glader,* and I write for a living. I love the act of communication and connection, and I believe in the power of talking to heal. I was lucky enough to live around the block from Nancy, and after what seemed like the eighth person to tell me I had to try to grab this comet of a woman, I managed to meet her. We immediately got each other, and I saw in her the kind of deep integrity that comes from helping others with the emotional questions right here, right now. She helped organize my very first book reading and was always there with encouragement and her special sauce of honesty and sass. Writing here is absolutely my pleasure.

You can learn about *Nowhere Hair,* my children's book now in its second printing (and available in Spanish as *¿Y el Pelo?*), on my website Nowhere Hair *(www.NowhereHair.com).*

Kelly Gallaher Greene was born on the East Coast in 1944 and raised on the West Coast. She has two beautiful daughters and three fabulous grandchildren, two girls and a boy. Kelly has spent a good part of her life studying transpersonal psychology and human behavior.

Allison W. Gryphon is a writer, filmmaker, and breast cancer fighter with a passion for story and an undying appetite for living life to the fullest. She currently works to make getting through the day-to-day of fighting cancer easier for people through her newly created network, The Why? Foundation.

Allison's directorial debut, the feature documentary *What the F@#- Is Cancer and Why Does Everybody Have It?*, rallied support from the Hollywood community. For the most part, Allison paid them with cookies. In association with the feature film, a collection of personal stories and programs focusing on specific cancers, treatments, and experiences will be released through a series of webisodes titled *The What? Series* that hit YouTube on November 20, 2014.

Her feature film *La Cucina*, for which she wrote the screenplay, won Best Picture at the Beloit International Film Festival and the Los Angeles Backlot Film Festival, as well as Best Screenplay at the Bragacine Festival International de Cinema in Portugal. Allison's first novel, the supernatural thriller entitled *Blood Moon*, is the first book in her Witches Moon Trilogy. In addition, Allison is stepping behind the camera once again to direct the feature punk rock documentary *Hong Kong Cafe*, about the notorious L.A. club.

The Why? Foundation (www.thewhyfoundation.org)

Susan Gubar revolutionized the study of literature by co-authoring the classic feminist text *The Madwoman in the Attic*, in 1979, followed by four powerful anthologies on women's literature. An acclaimed author and distinguished retired professor of English, Susan has recently turned her fierce talents to writing about ovarian cancer in her *Memoir of a Debulked Woman* (2012), and in "Living with Cancer" blogs for *The New York Times*. Susan received the Ivan Sandrof Lifetime Achievement Award of the National Book Critics Circle, along with her long-time collaborator Sandra M. Gilbert, in 2012. Her influence as a truth-teller continues to grow.

Dr. Kevin Haugh has been the retired Principal of Galvone N.S.

Limerick City, Ireland, since 2010. He was Assistant National Coordinator with Leadership Development for Schools 2005-2009, and is currently Coordinator of the Annual International Limerick & Clare Education Centres' Education Research Conference. In 2013, Haugh published *An Imperfect Storm* (Outside The Box Learning Resources, Naas, Co. Kildare, Ireland), which is available in paperback and Kindle editions.

Dagmar Herbstreuter was born in Germany in 1964. She moved to the San Francisco Bay Area in 1989, as part of a career-training program for eighteen months. Dagmar is still there, still learning. She has circled the globe in her field of work for the past twenty years, so she considers herself a global citizen. Dagmar loves yoga, anything creative—design, fashion, photography—and being in the great outdoors.

Hey guys, my name's *Jack Lagomarsino*. I'm a writer living and working in Los Angeles. I was in high school when my mom was diagnosed with breast cancer.

At that time, I needed her to know how sure I was that she'd be okay. I needed my dad to know that I had zero doubt in my mind that his wife would beat cancer and continue to be the wise, generous, and hilarious woman we loved and needed so much.

So I wrote a happy ending to the story she was living. It was the ending I truly believed in, and it was the ending we were lucky enough to live out.

Max Jennings, a graduate of the University of Southern California and a Minnesota native, currently works at Holden Village in the Cascades of North Central Washington State. He is a writer and train enthusiast.

Sophia Kercher calls herself a writer, dreamer, doer, and cancer eradication advocate. She is the editorial director of *Reimagine. me*, an online magazine and community and education program aimed at helping those who have been touched by cancer. Her articles and essays have been published in the *Los Angeles Times, Salon, LA Weekly,* and *Pasadena Magazine,* among other publications. She lives, writes, and dreams in Los Angeles, California.

Aenea M. Keyes—Before I was a cancer survivor, I thought of myself mainly in terms of "what I do"—as a classical violinist and international performer. During my illness, my focus moved toward staying close to home and living a healthy life. So I founded the San Francisco-based piano trio, MusicAEterna, which has seen me through years of illness and cancer recovery. MusicAEterna continues to perform established repertoire with our signature ChamberImprov, creating an artistic dialogue between music and visual art. Our new album, *Seasons, a Musical Dialogue,* was recorded at Skywalker Sound, and it celebrates life!
MusicAEterna (www.MusicAEternaUSA.com)

As a reporter with the San Joaquin News Service, *Les Mahler* covered the San Joaquin County Board of Supervisors from 2004 to 2006. Les is the founder of Stomp Out Cancer, an organization in northern California that funds research for a cure for pediatric cancer. It also helps families who are dealing with financial challenges due to their child's cancer battle.

Les wrote a poem which he thinks "says it all":

I am a cancer patient, not a victim;
as such, I am the same person I was before the cancer.
My spirit, sense of joy, unbridled passion for life,
sense of humor, dreams and goals
and aspirations to enjoy and do what I want
have not changed.
My love for friends and family did not fade or die away
and my joy in being with them still beats strong inside.
I still dance by the song of the rains,
still whisper to the moonlight,
still sing when the sun breaks the morning darkness
and laugh when my heart is filled with happiness.
I have not relinquished my dreams to any disease
And never will.
I have not given up on enjoying life to its fullest
And do not intend to do so.
I am still in love with life and always will be,
no matter what.
And each morning, I am thankful and feel blessed
that I can still greet the day
And see the sun rise above me;
Yes, I am a cancer patient like many others.
And no matter what we go through
We are not victims and never will be.

Russ Messing—I am a psychologist, a poet, a committed father and husband, and Nancy's long-time friend (fifty-seven years, plus or minus). Nancy's project matters to me because I believe she shines a warm and optimistic light over the scourge of cancer. Her story is one of resilience, unabashed optimism, courage, and commitment. It has been an honor to walk beside her.

Alexander Niles was diagnosed with stage IV gastric cancer in the fall of 2013, at age thirty. He is the founder of CureWear (www.mycurewear.com), a lifestyle apparel line designed to provide comfort for cancer patients during treatment, while inspiring their friends and family. He is also writing a book geared towards younger cancer battlers, that sets forth his positive, activist approach to fighting the illness.

Alexander holds an undergraduate degree from Drexel University, where he was a Division 1 scholarship athlete, and a graduate degree from Fordham University. His work has been featured in *The New York Times, Huffington Post,* and *Psychology Today.*

Linda Novack, M.A., is a Master Certified Coach, workshop facilitator, and corporate consultant. She has been exploring and stretching into new possibilities and the expansion of consciousness for over thirty years. As the principal of Novack & Associates—a consulting firm specializing in performance excellence through coaching, organization development, and training—Linda has worked with individuals to achieve success and fulfillment in all aspects of their lives and to effectively navigate through life's transitions. She specializes in working with women, facilitating growth in their professional and personal lives.

Linda loves to discover life's unfolding mysteries and joys through travel, meditation, hiking, painting, yoga, and the

community of good friends and family.
Novack and Associates (www.novackandassociates.com)

Nancy Novack—On the day of the tenth anniversary of my diagnosis, I shouted out loud, "Follow your bliss. Follow your heart."

If I were to be true to that, I would sell my fabulous house in Mill Valley, pack up my two dogs, Lucy and Bozo, and my African grey parrot Floyd, say good-bye to my many friends of forty and fifty years of togetherness, say good-bye to the beauty and grandeur of the Bay Area, leave my Berkeley hippie history of which I am so proud, and move in with my Cowboy (he is really not a cowboy but I love the fantasy that he is—we have no horses) in Austin, where the mean temperature is over 100 degrees half the year, and everyone talks fairly funny, and I will never ever have a girlfriend like I do in California. And, if you know me at all, that decision took years. I totally angst-ed day and night.

Was I well enough, sane enough to leave my sacred sanctuary—my blue and silver house with the purple stairs and the white rose gardens? I love so many things about my California life—my truly inspiring nonprofits Nancy's List and Nancy's Club, and all the courageous grown-ups and children I adore, and my brave psychotherapy clients, and the extraordinary relationships in the Bay Area cancer community that I have formed through Nancy's List. I couldn't imagine leaving the nearness to my Los Angeles family and my super grandchildren and, of course, could I exist without all my lovely lady friends? I knew I would miss the sailing, the horseback riding, Stinson Beach, my Marin and San Francisco life. How could I trade my fabulous restaurants for breakfast tacos? How could I leave the wacko San Francisco politics and ever understand or accept the ever more so wacko Texas politics?

During my cancer journey, I learned to live and love with an open heart. To say yes. And definitely, to go for pleasure. So I did it. I put on my fabulous cowgirl hat, my black patent leather cowgirl boots. I will follow my passion and my purpose and hopefully bring Nancy's List to Austin.

Austin is cool and my guy is totally cool.

And I am happy . . . extraordinarily happy.

Thank you to everyone who rooted for me to be healthy and happy and to the many angels who pointed the way.

Nancy's List (www.nancyslist.org)

Laurie Hessen Pomeranz, MFT, lives in San Francisco with her husband and son Jack. She is a high school counselor, Stella & Dot jewelry stylist, baseball enthusiast, singer in a tot-rock band, cancer survivor, and grateful mama.

Stella & Dot (www.stelladot.com/lauriepomeranz)

I'm *Bonnie Powers,* managing director for Hatch (www.hatchsf.com), a creative agency in San Francisco, as well as the brand director of Jeffrey Levin (www.jeffreylevin.com), my husband's fine jewelry collection. With a family business, in addition to a full-time job, my work life is busy. When my health was at stake, recently, and with limited examples to learn from, I realized that I could help others through my journey by documenting the research, surgery prep, and recovery from cancer. Being transparent through my blog BRCA2: In This Together (www.brca2gether.wordpress.com), and supporting projects like *I Am with*

You, gives me the hope that no one goes through cancer alone.

Holly Pruett is a certified Life-Cycle Celebrant and Home Funeral Guide, and founder of PDX Death Café in Portland, Oregon.

Leslie Purchase was a former physician and mother of three kids, ages four, two, and six months, when she was diagnosed with triple negative breast cancer at age thirty-two. In the five years since then, she has raised her children, survived the brain cancer diagnosis of her youngest child, at age two, and she recently started a company to encourage baseline concussion testing for everyone. Leslie's desire to give hope to newly diagnosed patients is rooted in her knowledge that there is hope and life after cancer. Her family is a wonderful example of that.

Rachel Naomi Remen, M.D., is Clinical Professor of Family and Community Medicine at UCSF School of Medicine, and Founder and Director of the Institute for the Study of Health and Illness at Commonweal. She is one of the best-known of the early pioneers of Holistic and Integrative Medicine. As a medical educator, therapist, and teacher, Rachel has enabled many thousands of physicians and other health professionals to work from the heart, and thousands of patients to remember their power to heal. Her groundbreaking curriculum for medical students, The Healer's Art, is taught in ninety of America's medical schools and medical schools in seven countries abroad.

This master storyteller and observer of life has published two bestselling books, *Kitchen Table Wisdom* and *My Grandfather's Blessings,* which have sold more than a million copies and are translated into twenty-three languages. Rachel has had Crohn's

disease for more than sixty years, and her work is a unique blend of the wisdom, strength, and experience of both doctor and patient.
Rachel Naomi Remen, M.D. (www.rachelremen.com)
Remembering the Heart of Medicine (www.theheartofmedicine.org)
Ishi (www.ishiprograms.org)

Editor *Barbara K. Richardson* earned her M.F.A. in creative writing and literary editing from Eastern Washington University. Her novel *Tributary* (2012) won the Utah Book Award in Fiction and was a WILLA Award Finalist in Historical Fiction. Her upcoming anthology, *Dirt: A Love Story* (2015), extols the virtues of dirt. She loves great books and open landscapes.
Barbara K. Richardson (www.barbarakrichardson.com)
Dirt: A Love Story (www.dirtalovestory.com)

Elana Rosenbaum, MS, LICSW, has been a leader in the clinical application of mindfulness meditation to cancer care for over twenty-five years. She has authored *Here for Now: Living Well with Cancer through Mindfulness* (Satya House, 2007), and *Being Well (Even When You're Sick)* (Shambala, 2012), the basis of many workshops and audio-CDs with guided meditations. In 1995, she was diagnosed with non-Hodgkin's lymphoma and subsequently underwent stem cell transplantation. Her ability to thrive and embody mindfulness in the face of adversity led to the development of a mindfulness-based intervention for bone marrow transplant patients at the University of Massachusetts Medical Center, Emory University, and Dana Farber Cancer Institute.

She is adjunct faculty at the renowned Stress Reduction Clinic at the University of Massachusetts Medical School, where

she worked directly with Jon Kabat-Zinn as one of the founding teachers. Elana has a private practice in psychotherapy in Worcester, Massachusetts, and is a sought-after teacher, speaker, workshop leader, and research consultant.
Mindful Living (www.mindfulliving.com)

Gabrielle Roth chose dance as her profession at age seven — or did dance choose her? Loving ballet, gypsy dancing, yoga, and all types of movement, Gabrielle developed a structure for dance as a transformative process at Esalen Institute. This began her world-famous 5Rhythms program which now has hundreds of teachers worldwide. Her book *Sweat Your Prayers* (Tarcher, 1998) outlines the power of dance to lead us "back into the garden, back to the earth, whole and healed, spirit and flesh reunited." A dancer, actress, director, and performer, Roth produced over twenty albums of rhythmical musical bliss with her band, the Mirrors.

The Moving Center in New York City, which she founded, continues to teach Gabrielle's techniques for unlocking body rhythms as a way to heighten consciousness through dance. In 5Rhythms, "movement is the medicine, the meditation and the metaphor."
5Rhythms (www.5rhythms.com)

Leslie Roth has been performing caretaking tasks for years for her mother, her husband, her friends and cousins. She is a naturally caring person. But she does not do this professionally. She is a professional artist, working as a painter, ceramic sculptor, and illustrator in San Francisco. You can see her work on her website.
Leslie Roth (www.LeslieRothArt.com)

Benjamin Rubenstein began writing his memoir, *Twice: How I Became a Cancer-Slaying Super Man Before I Turned 21*, while attending college at the University of Virginia where he also began blogging on Cancerslayerblog (www.cancerslayerblog.com). *Twice* was published in 2010, and a year later he began writing his next book for kids, *Secrets of the Cancer-Slaying Super Man*. Before his books were published, Rubenstein never discussed his journeys with cancer, though he now feels that sharing his story has been among his most rewarding experiences. This is his passion and why he chose to participate in *I Am with You*.

John Smith — I was sixty-one years old when diagnosed with multiple myeloma, an incurable blood cancer. Shocked? Yes. Depressed? No. My wife and I set to work to understand what the cancer was all about. Most online queries gave grim statistical prognoses. However, I also discovered the blogs of actual patients, some of whom painted a different picture. Due to their writing, I learned that hope for managing this disease was possible. I attribute the effort of other patients to inspiring me to write of my own journey and, here I am, seven years later, passing the torch of hope onto others.
Good Blood, Bad Blood (www.goodbloodbadblood.wordpress.com)

Annie Sprinkle, Ph.D., was a New York City prostitute and porn star for twenty years, then morphed into an artist and sexologist. She has passionately explored sexuality for forty years, sharing her experiences through making her own unique brand of feminist sex films, writing, art making, and performance. Currently, Annie is a mover and shaker in the "ecosex movement," committed

to making environmentalism more sexy, fun, and diverse.
Annie Sprinkle (www.anniesprinkle.org)
Sex Ecology (www.sexecology.org)

Terri White Tate, RN, MS, is a keynote speaker and storyteller
whose life and voice were threatened by two bouts of oral cancer from which she had a 2 percent chance of survival. But
her sense of humor was never in danger. Terri's hilarious solo
show, *Shopping as a Spiritual Path,* chronicles life's challenges
and triumphs. Audiences across the country have been moved
to laughter, tears, and standing ovations by her powerful performances. She is putting the finishing touches on the memoir
of her cancer journey, with an introduction by Anne Lamott.
Because Terri teaches storytelling with an emphasis on speaking
from the soul, she knows the tremendous healing power of sharing our stories, and so is delighted to be part of *I Am with You.*
Terri White Tate (www.territate.com)

Shariann Tom is the Founder and President of The Cancer
Journey, which blends two turning points for Shariann: surviving
four bouts of lymphoma and one bout with a gastrointestinal
stromal tumor (GIST), and making life coaching her profession. The profound contrast between facing cancer without a
coach and a cancer journey with a coach inspired Shariann to
start a movement dedicated to cancer patients, caregivers, and
survivors. "I was in a state of panic and coaching allowed me to
feel I had power." Hence, the "Panic to Powerful Program" and
Cancer Journey Coaching were born. "I want this for everyone
who is touched by cancer," says Shariann. "It gives people access
to true healing."

Shariann's sixteen years of coaching and coach training, combined with her sixteen years in corporate America in business management and sales and marketing, allow her the balance needed to run and operate an innovative company. Shariann is regularly asked to speak to cancer support centers and health conferences across the country. She lives in the San Francisco Bay Area where she can be near her family, both nuclear and extended.

The Cancer Journey (www.thecancerjourney.com)

Marcy Westerling—I am a longtime community organizer with a passion for justice, and I founded the Rural Organizing Project in 1992. Derailed by a stage IV ovarian cancer diagnosis in spring 2010, I have stayed in treatment since then. I strive to embrace "livingly dying." I hope that by being game for cutting-edge treatments, I will have more time to find the sweet spots of thriving while terminally ill. I am currently in my seventh line of treatment and think of it as my full-time (and least exciting) job.

Livingly Dying (www.LivinglyDying.com)

Lisa Marie Wilson was born in Michigan to an Elvis impersonator and a nurse on welfare, but currently resides in Los Angeles, not on welfare. She writes and produces for both TV and online. Lisa Marie blogs regularly for *The Huffington Post*, and has appeared on the TV show *Ten Things I Hate About You*. She recently starred in a TV pilot titled *Over the Hill*, with Robert Wagner and Tim Conway.

Lisa Marie's book, *Traveling Daisy: A Generational Cancer Story of Disease and Dysfunction*, asks the question, "Did my chaotic life cause my cancer?" A number-one bestseller in cancer books on Amazon, this e-book donates all its proceeds to benefit cancer research. Lisa Marie is the fifth generation of her family to be diagnosed with the disease. Her family has dealt with breast, colon, melanoma, carcinoid, and thyroid cancers. She wants to help people, and feels blessed when they say that something she wrote made a difference to their attitudes about cancer.

Traveling Daisy (www.TravelingDaisy.com)

CREDITS

"You Are Not Your Cancer" by Paul Brenner.
Published in *Stand Up to Cancer* newsletter.

"How to Woo a Doctor" by Aisling Carroll.
Published in *The Huffington Post*, 11/8/2011.

"Why My BFFs Are My Chore Whores" by Aisling Carroll.
Published in *The Huffington Post*, 12/9/2011.

"Got Cancer: Now What?" by Paige Davis.
Published in *The Huffington Post*, 5/18/2014.

"I Bought a Peacock" by Paige Davis.
Published in *The Huffington Post*, 6/9/2014.

"Divatude" by Daphne D. Evans. Daphne is Founder of
Heaven's Door Cancer Foundation, a national wellness spa
treatment and advocacy program for women with cancer and
advanced life-threatening illnesses.

"I Watched My Mom Reinvent Herself" by Sophia Kercher. Published in *Reimagine.me*, 3/26/2014.

"Fear" by Alexander Niles. Published in *Psychology Today*, May 19, 2014. It also appeared as "What is Fear?" in *The Huffington Post*, May 19, 2014.

"My Cancer and My Son" by Laurie Hessen Pomeranz. Published in *The Mother Company* (online), May 12, 2011 and in *The Day My Nipple Fell Off and Other Stories of Survival, Solidarity, and Sass: a BAYS Anthology*, 2013.

"Bigger than Prince" by Bonnie Powers. Published as "This is My Truth—Cancer Trauma & BRCA Recovery" on her website BRCA2: In This Together (*brca2gether.wordpress.com*).

"Two Tiny Green Blades of Grass" by Rachel Naomi Remen. A version of the story appeared in *Kitchen Table Wisdom*, published by Riverhead Press, 1996. Dr. Remen has retold the story for this work.

"Coping with Cancer" by Elana Rosenbaum. Published in *Mindful* magazine.

"To My Next Thirty Cancer-Free Years" by Benjamin Rubenstein. Copyright © Benjamin Rubenstein.

"Livingly Dying" by Marcy Westerling.

Published in *Yes! Magazine*, Fall 2014
(www.yesmagazine.org/issues/the-end-of-poverty/livingly-dying).

"Fighting Terminal Cancer With Life" by Lisa Marie Wilson.
Published in *The Huffington Post*, 8/18/2014.

ACKNOWLEDGMENTS

To Theo Gund, my sweet friend, who made it all happen, and whose dedication, understanding, compassion, and enthusiasm inspired me and gave me the courage to embrace so many stories of hope and struggle.

To Barbara Richardson, who did it all as my awesome editor, and who understood the need for truth and beauty. She brought to the collection harmony, honesty, knowledge, precision, and rare intuition.

To Jake Messing and Corrin Acome, who indulged me with their magnificent artistry for the cover and the interior design, and sighed with each of my defective personality indecisions.

To the extraordinary authors who revealed their inner truths, their challenges, and reached out their hands of support and their hearts filled with love and grace to everyone who walks the cancer walk, struts the cancer strut. Bless you and please stay well.

To Dr. Branimir Sikic, my oncologist at Stanford, who taught me the inevitable power of human connection in the healing process.

And to my family and friends and loved ones and all the people I never met but who cheered me on . . . who stayed beside me every step . . . who brought meaning to my journey, who opened my heart and let the love flow in.

To my huge A Team who always knew I would make it.

To my daddy, who always wanted to help me, and to my mom, who refused to believe I ever had cancer.

And to my amazing parrot Floyd . . . who walked like a pigeon into my room when I was so sleepy that I couldn't raise my head . . . and said, "Do you want to sing?"

And to my children, Steven and Carrie, and their children, Sebastian and Alexandra, who made me really want to live a long, long time.

And to my beloved, David. We delight in each other.